The Glucose Re
Revoluti

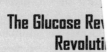

■

"For decades we've known that success in athletics is based not only on how athletes train, but also on what they eat. Now *The Glucose Revolution* provides scientifically based nutritional advice to help athletes achieve peak performance and answers their many questions about what and when to eat before, during, and after competition. It clearly explains that eating high-carbohydrate foods when in training is not enough—the glycemic index must also be considered."
—JOE FRIEL, author of *The Triathlete's Training Bible* and *The Cyclist's Training Bible*

"Forget *Sugar Busters*. Forget *The Zone*. If you want the real scoop on how carbohydrates and sugar affect your body, read this book by the world's leading researchers on the subject. It's the authoritative, last word on choosing foods to control your blood sugar."
—JEAN CARPER, best-selling author of *Miracle Brain, Miracle Cures, Stop Aging Now!* and *Food—Your Miracle Medicine*

"The glycemic index is a useful tool which may have a broad spectrum of applications, from the maintenance of fuel supply during exercise to the control of blood glucose levels in diabetics. Low glycemic index foods may prove to have beneficial health effects for all of us in the long-term. *The Glucose Revolution* is a user-friendly, easy-to-read overview of all that you need to know about the glycemic index. This book represents a balanced account of the importance of the glycemic index based on sound scientific evidence."

—JAMES HILL, Ph.D., Director, Center for Human Nutrition, University of Colorado Health Sciences Center

"The concept of the glycemic index has been distorted and bastardized by popular writers and diet gurus. Here, at last, is a book that explains what we know about the glycemic index and its importance in designing a diet for optimum health. Carbohydrates are not all bad. Read the good news about pasta and even—believe it or not—sugar!"

—ANDREW WEIL, M.D., University of Arizona College of Medicine, author of *Spontaneous Healing* and *8 Weeks to Optimum Health*

"*The Glucose Revolution* is nutrition science for the 21st century. Clearly written, it gives the scientific rationale for why all carbohydrates are not created equal. It is a practical guide for both professionals and patients. The food suggestions and recipes are exciting and tasty."

—RICHARD N. PODELL, M.D., M.P.H., Clinical Professor, Department of Family Medicine, UMDNJ-Robert Wood Johnson Medical School, and co-author of *The G-Index Diet: The Missing Link That Makes Permanent Weight Loss Possible*

The GLUCOSE *Revolution*

POCKET GUIDE TO
SPORTS NUTRITION

HELEN O'CONNOR, B.Sc., DIP. N.D., PH.D.

JENNIE BRAND-MILLER, PH.D.

THOMAS M.S. WOLEVER, M.D., PH.D.

STEPHEN COLAGIURI, M.D.

KAYE FOSTER-POWELL, M. NUTR. & DIET.

ADAPTED BY
JOHANNA BURANI, M.S., R.D., C.D.E.
AND LINDA RAO, M.ED.

■

MARLOWE & COMPANY
NEW YORK

Published by
Marlowe & Company
841 Broadway, 4th Floor
New York, NY 10003

This book is not intended to replace the services of a physician or dietitian. Any application of the recommendations set forth in the following pages is at the reader's discretion. The reader should consult with his or her own physician or dietitian concerning the recommendations in this book.

First published in Australia in 1997 in somewhat different form under the title *Pocket Guide to the G.I. Factor and Sports Nutrition* by Hodder Headline Australia Pty Limited.

This edition is published by arrangement with Hodder Headline Australia Pty Limited.

Library of Congress Cataloging-in-Publication Data
Pocket guide to the G.I. factor and sports nutrition.
    The glucose revolution pocket guide to sports nutrition / by Jennie Brand-Miller . . . [et al.].
        p. cm.
    Previously pub. as: Pocket guide to the G.I. factor and sports nutrition. Sydney : Hodder & Stoughton, 1997.
    ISBN 1-56924-676-9
    1. Athletes—Nutrition.   2. Glycemic index.   I. Brand-Miller, Janette, 1952-   II. Title.

TX361.A8 P63 2000
613.2'024'796—dc21

                                                            99-042188

9 8 7 6 5 4 3 2 1
Designed by Pauline Neuwirth, Neuwirth & Associates, Inc.
Distributed by Publishers Group West
Manufactured in the United States of America

CONTENTS

PREFACE

---

*T*he *Glucose Revolution* is the definitive, all-in-one guide to the glycemic index. Now we have written this pocket guide to show you how the glycemic index (G.I.) can help you to enhance your sports performance—whether you're a weekend warrior or a serious athlete.

The Glucose Revolution Pocket Guide to Sports Nutrition offers more in-depth information about using the glycemic index to boost your athletic performance than we had room to include in *The Glucose Revolution.* Much new information appears in this book that is not in *The Glucose Revolution,* including the questions most frequently asked by athletes about the glycemic index, recommendations about what to eat before a competition, during an event, and for a quick recovery, and success stories profiling athletes who have gained the winning edge by eating low—and high—G.I. foods at the appropriate times.

This book has been written to be read alongside *The Glucose Revolution,* so in the event you haven't already consulted that book, please be sure to do so, for a more comprehensive discussion of the glycemic index and all its uses.

Chapter 1

HOW THIS BOOK CAN HELP YOU

*S*ports nutrition is a new and dynamic science dedicated to unraveling the key nutrition factors that boost sports performance. What you eat does make a difference to your performance. The trick is getting into the right eating routine, keeping up to date and ignoring the confusing nutrition myths that abound.

This book looks at a new key factor: the glycemic index (or G.I.). Australian researchers were the first to see the potential in applying the glycemic index to athletes' diets to enhance sports performance, and now trainers, registered dietitians and athletes the world over are using the glycemic index to give them a competitive edge.

WHAT IS THE GLYCEMIC INDEX?

The glycemic index of foods is simply a ranking of foods based on their immediate effect on blood sugar levels. To make a fair comparison, all foods are compared with a reference food such as pure glucose and are tested in equivalent carbohydrate amounts.

Originally, research into the glycemic index of foods was inspired by the desire to identify the best foods for people with diabetes. But scientists are now discovering that G.I. values have implications for everyone, including athletes and other very active people.

Today we know the glycemic index of hundreds of different food items—both generic and name brand—that have been tested following a standardized testing method. The tables in Chapter 19 give the glycemic index of a range of common foods, including many tested at the University of Toronto and the University of Sydney.

The glycemic index ranks carbohydrate foods on the speed at which they enter the bloodstream. The faster a blood sugar response appears in the bloodstream after eating a food, the higher its ranking or its glycemic index. The longer it takes to observe a blood sugar response, the lower the glycemic index.

Some of the lowest G.I. carbohydrate foods are legumes (including soybeans, baked beans and lentils). These enter the bloodstream slowly and have a very low glycemic index (soybeans have a glycemic index of 18).

This guide shows you how to use the glycemic index in your own diet to boost your sports performance. When you pop this pocket book into your training bag, you'll have:

- a quick quiz to help you assess your current eating habits
- refueling tips at your fingertips
- case studies that provide you with fun, easy and practical ways to eat your way to better performance
- G.I. tables of foods, including sports drinks, plus their fat and carbohydrate count

■

WHAT YOU EAT DOES MAKE A DIFFERENCE
TO YOUR SPORTS PERFORMANCE.

■

Chapter 2

IS YOUR DIET FIT FOR PEAK PERFORMANCE?

---

*D*o you think your current diet supplies you with the nutrients you need to perform at your best? Let's put it to the test. Take the following diet fitness quiz and see how well you score. It's a good idea to use this quiz regularly to pick up on areas where you may need to improve your diet.

1. Circle "Yes" or "No" below each quiz item.

Eating patterns
- I eat at least 3 meals a day with no longer than 5 hours in between
  Yes / No

Carbohydrate checker
- I eat at least 4 slices of bread each day (1 roll = 2 slices of bread)
  Yes / No
- I eat at least 1 cup of breakfast cereal each day or an extra slice of bread
  Yes / No
- I usually eat 2 or more pieces of fruit each day
  Yes / No
- I eat at least 5 different vegetables or have a large salad most days
  Yes / No
- I include carbohydrates like pasta, rice and potato in my diet each day
  Yes / No

Protein checker
- I eat at least 1 and usually 2 servings of meat or meat alternatives (poultry, seafood, eggs, dried peas, beans or nuts) each day
  Yes / No

Fat checker
- I spread butter or margarine thinly on bread or use none at all
  Yes / No
- I eat fried food no more than once per week
  Yes / No
- I use polyunsaturated or monounsaturated oil (canola or olive) for cooking. (Circle yes if you never fry in oil or fat)
  Yes / No
- I avoid oil-based dressings on salads
  Yes / No
- I use reduced fat or low fat dairy products
  Yes / No

- I cut the fat off meat and take the skin off chicken
  Yes / *No*
- I eat fatty snacks such as chocolate, chips, biscuits or rich desserts/cakes etc. no more than twice a week
  Yes / *No*
- I eat fast or takeout food no more than once per week
  Yes / *No*

Iron checker

- I eat lean red meat at least 3 times per week or 2 servings of white meat daily or for vegetarians, include at least 1 or 2 cups of dried peas and beans (such as lentils, soy beans, chickpeas) daily
  Yes / *No*
- I include a vitamin C source with meals based on bread, cereals, fruit and vegetables to assist the iron absorption in these plant sources of iron
  Yes / *No*

Calcium checker

- I eat at least 3 servings of dairy food or soy milk alternative each day (1 serving = 8 ounces milk or fortified soy milk; 1 ounce slice of hard cheese; 8 ounces yogurt)
  Yes / *No*

Fluids

- I drink fluids regularly before, during and after exercise
  Yes / *No*

Alcohol
- When I drink alcohol, I usually drink no more than is recommended for the safe driving limit (Circle "Yes" if you don't drink alcohol)
  Yes / No

2. Score 1 point for every "Yes" answer

Scoring scale
18–20: Excellent
15–17: Room for improvement
12–14: Just made it
0–12: Poor

Note: *Very* active people will need to eat more breads, cereals and fruit than we have outlined on this quiz, but to stay healthy no one should be eating less. (Adapted from *The Taste of Fitness* by Helen O'Connor and Donna Hay)

Chapter 3

SPORTS NUTRITION IN A NUTSHELL

To perform at its best, your body needs the right type of fuel. No matter what your sport, carbohydrates are the best fuel for you! High carbohydrate foods help enhance stamina and prevent fatigue. These types of food include breakfast cereals, bread, rice, pasta, fruit and vegetables (especially starchy vegetables like new potatoes, corn and dried peas and beans). Sugars found in table sugar, honey, jam and candy are also useful sources of carbohydrate for active people.

LOW FAT EATING

Fats are an essential part of your diet. A low to moderate fat intake helps active people maintain a lean physique. But eating the *best types of fat* and avoiding excessive fat intake is important for good health as well as best performance. The best types of fats for cooking include the monounsaturated fats such as olive and canola oil and the polyunsaturated fats such as sunflower and safflower oil. Watch out for the saturated fats found in many fast foods, as well as butter, cream and the visible fat on meat.

It's never to late to start reducing the amount of fat in your diet. Here's how:

- cut the fat off meat (or use lean cuts)
- remove the skin from chicken
- use minimal amounts of fat in cooking, or substitute with vegetable sprays
- use nonstick cookware

The amount of fat you need depends on your daily fuel requirements. For good health and weight maintenance we have included the following general guidelines. (5 g fat is equivalent to about 1 teaspoon mono- or polyunsaturated oil.)

Low fat diets	30 to 40 g fat per day
Most women and children	30 to 50 g fat per day
Most men	40 to 60 g fat per day
Teenagers and active adults	70 g fat per day
Larger and very active athletes/workers	80 to 100 g fat per day

Fat is a seemingly invisible ingredient in many foods. Use a fat counter to help you identify some of the sources of fat in your diet. Keep a food record for a week and calculate your personal fat intake using the counter. It may surprise you! (Comprehensive fat counters are readily available from bookstores and supermarkets.) To lend a hand, we have also included a fat counter in the A–Z of Foods table in this pocket guide starting on page 94.

ARE YOU REALLY CHOOSING LOW FAT?

There's a trick to food labels that it is worth being aware of when shopping for low fat foods. These food labeling specification guidelines were enacted by the United States Department of Agriculture (USDA) in 1994:

Free: Contains a tiny or insignificant amount of fat, cholesterol, sodium, sugar or calories; less than 0.5 grams (g) of fat per serving.
Low fat: Contains no more than 3 g of fat per serving.
Reduced/Less/Fewer: These diet products must contain 25 percent less of a nutrient to calories than the regular product.
Light/Lite: These diet products contain ⅓ fewer calories than, or ½ the fat of, the original product.
Lean: Meats claiming this contain less than 10 g of fat, 4 g of saturated fat, and 95 milligrams (mg) of cholesterol per serving.
Extra lean: These meats have less than 5 g of fat, 2 g of saturated fat, 95 mg of cholesterol.

■

A BALANCED DIET
CONTAINS A WIDE
VARIETY OF LOW FAT FOODS.

■

DON'T FORGET PROTEIN

Athletes in heavy training have increased protein needs. Protein balance depends on the individual, but you generally need at least 2 or 3 servings a day. Some athletes forget to include enough protein in their diets, while body builders often consume more protein than their bodies need. Good sources of protein include lean meat, poultry, fish and seafood, eggs, milk, cheese and yogurt. Dried peas, beans and nuts are the best vegetable sources. Bread and cereals provide smaller, but still useful, amounts of protein.

FLUIDS

The human body is 70 percent water. During exercise you lose some of this water as sweat. If you don't replace it, you will become dehydrated and your body will overheat—like a car without water in its radiator.

- Small fluid losses decrease performance.
- Large fluid losses can result in dehydration and are life-threatening!

During exercise, thirst isn't a good indicator of how much fluid your body needs, so don't use that as your guide! Be sure to drink more than your thirst dictates. Every pound lost during exercise approximates 1 pint of sweat losses to be replaced.

■

DURING EXERCISE,
THIRST IS NOT A GOOD INDICATOR OF YOUR FLUID NEEDS.

■

WHAT TO DRINK DURING EXERCISE

It's hard to know exactly what to drink when you're working out, because there are so many options! From water to sports drinks to fruit juice, here are some guidelines to help quench your thirst:

- **Water** replaces lost fluids adequately in many situations.
- **Sports and electrolyte drinks** are absorbed into the bloodstream faster than water. In addition to replacing carbohydrates and electrolytes, they taste good, which encourages you to drink more. (See Chapter 10 on page 47 for more on sports drinks.) The A–Z of Foods (Chapter 19 on page 105) gives the glycemic index of sports drinks, such as Gatorade and Sportsplus. Please note that this does not refer to sport supplement drinks such as Ensure Light or Super Shake, which are liquid meals.
- **Soft drinks or fruit juice** empty from the stomach more slowly than sports drinks or water and aren't suitable fluid replacers during exercise.

Note: Be careful with caffeine-containing beverages while exercising. The caffeine increases urine production, which can make you dehydrated.

■

ADEQUATE FLUID REPLACEMENT
DURING EXERCISE ENHANCES PERFORMANCE
AND PREVENTS HEAT STRESS.

■

SPECIAL NUTRIENT CONSIDERATIONS

Of course, everyone—athletes and non-athletes alike—needs to make sure they're eating right and getting adequate amounts of important nutrients. But athletes, laborers and avid exercisers need to be especially careful to take in the appropriate amounts of vitamins, minerals and other nutrients to perform better and longer, without ill effects.

Iron

Iron deficiency is common in athletes, particularly female athletes, vegetarians and those participating in strenuous training programs, such as endurance athletes. Many athletes don't consume adequate iron in their daily diets and may take in too much caffeine or tannin (in tea) that binds up the available iron and reduces its absorption. The best sources of iron are red meats and liver. Plant sources contain lower amounts of iron, and the iron isn't absorbed as well.

BEST SOURCES OF IRON

(ranked from highest to lowest):
* **** Red meats and liver
* *** White meats and seafood
* ** Dried peas and beans (baked beans, soy beans)
* * Bread, cereals and some vegetables

Did you know?

Including vitamin C rich fruits and vegetables in a meal improves the absorption or iron from plant sources (e.g. bread, cereals, vegetables, fruit).

Calcium

Calcium is important for bone development in young people and for bone maintenance in adults. Getting enough calcium and participating in weight-bearing exercise throughout life is essential to build—then maintain—optimal bone strength for both males and females.

■

CALCIUM IS IMPORTANT FOR BONE DEVELOPMENT IN THE YOUNG AND FOR BONE MAINTENANCE IN ADULTS.

■

In females, regular strenuous exercise, usually accompanied by factors such as fat loss, strict dieting or stress, can precipitate menstrual cycle interruptions. An irregular or absent menstrual cycle may result in a reduced level of the hormone estrogen, which is vital for maintaining calcium levels in bone and for enhancing calcium absorption. If you have experienced menstrual irregularities for longer than six months, you should see a doctor to help determine the cause. Athletes with very infrequent or absent menstrual cycles should have extra calcium in the range of 1000 to 1500 mg a day. This won't prevent bone loss, but may help to slow down the rate of loss.

NUTRITIONAL SUPPLEMENTS

Companies spend lots of money promoting nutritional supplements for active people and athletes. Just watch out for supplements with no scientific basis to the claims. If in doubt, ask a sports dietitian for help. (See page 108 for information on locating a registered dietitian near you.) Some supplements are beneficial in certain circumstances.

- **You may need iron or calcium supplements** if you consume inadequate amounts of these minerals or if you have a deficiency.
- **You might also benefit from supplements such as sports drinks, liquid meals and carbohydrate loaders,** not because they provide anything magical, but because they package energy and carbohydrate in a convenient and easy-to-consume form. They're especially useful to athletes who need an easily digested fuel on the run.
- **Sports bars and carbohydrate gels** (available in sports and bike shops) are in a similar category to sports drinks.
- **Herbal supplements, amino acids and fat burners:** Unfortunately, solid evidence for these supplements is lacking. In many cases, scientific studies have shown absolutely no effect.
- **Always make sure that any supplements you take are safe and drug free.** Some herbal supplements have actually caused some athletes to register "positive" on drug tests. Check with your sport's governing body to make sure the herb or medicine that you're taking is approved.

COMPETITION EATING

Eating for competing is discussed in detail later in this book. Look under the following topics:

- Pre-competition meal guidelines (page 42)
- The case for low G.I. foods (page 22)

- Glycogen loading (page 40)
- Recovery after exercise (page 52)
- The case for high G.I. foods (page 51)
- Refueling during an event (page 47)

If you want to find out about eating for competing in greater depth, consult a sports dietitian. (To locate an R.D. near you, see the contact information on page 108.)

■

WHETHER YOU ARE ONE OF THE ELITE OR A WEEKEND WARRIOR, THE RIGHT DIET CAN GIVE YOU THE WINNING EDGE.

■

Chapter 4

ENERGY-CHARGE YOUR BODY WITH CARBOHYDRATE

Carbohydrate circulates in your body as glucose in the blood (blood sugar) and is stored as glycogen in the liver and muscles. When glycogen stores are depleted, fatigue sets in and performance suffers. Your body uses glucose to fuel movement and activity. Just as high-speed cars require regular gasoline fill-ups, active bodies need a regular supply of carbohydrate to fill up glycogen stores.

Carbohydrate is the human body's favorite energy source for physical activity—especially for high intensity exercise. But your body's carbohydrate stores are small and need regular replenishing, generally every four to five hours.

Athletes feel tired and lethargic when they don't consume enough carbohydrate to meet their daily needs. When this happens and the glycogen in the muscles is depleted, fatigue sets in. That's when your muscles feel heavy and your pace slows. "Hitting the wall," an expression used by endurance athletes, describes the feeling when glycogen stores are almost exhausted.

■

ACTIVE BODIES NEED A REGULAR SUPPLY OF CARBOHYDRATE TO FILL UP THEIR GLYCOGEN STORES.

■

LOW BLOOD SUGAR OR "HYPOGLYCEMIA"

People who work out can also experience a type of fatigue related to the carbohydrate levels in their blood. It is possible for your muscle glycogen levels to be adequate while the blood sugar levels controlled by the liver, fall. Low blood sugar (also known as "hypoglycemia") occurs when you exercise in the morning before eating, or exercise hard after skipping a meal.

■

TO MAINTAIN ENERGY LEVELS, ATHLETES MUST CONSUME ENOUGH CARBOHYDRATE TO KEEP PACE WITH THEIR MUSCLE GLYCOGEN NEEDS AND KEEP UP A REGULAR INTAKE OF CARBOHYDRATE TO MAINTAIN BLOOD SUGAR LEVELS.

■

EARLY MORNING EXERCISE

If you exercise strenuously early in the morning, it's a good idea to have some carbohydrate before training or take some with you to have on the run. Most people have enough liver glycogen to fuel low intensity, short duration (less than one hour) exercise sessions. If you simply want to delay eating until after your light early morning walk, it's not a problem. However, eating before and/or during a strenuous cycling session makes good sense!

THREE EASY STEPS TO ESTIMATE YOUR DAILY CARBOHYDRATE NEEDS

It's difficult to put an exact figure on anyone's carbohydrate needs. Use the table on pages 32–33 as a rough guide and ask a sports dietitian for help if you're unsure.

Step 1. Weigh yourself naked or in minimal clothing in kilograms. To do this, multiply your weight in pounds by 2.2. (Remember: no shoes or belts with heavy buckles!).

Step 2. Multiply your body weight by your activity level factor (see table on pages 32–33). This total gives you the **target carbohydrate intake in grams** that you must consume each day to meet your carbohydrate needs.

Step 3. Keep a food record for a few days and calculate your carbohydrate intake (use a carbohydrate counter such as the one at the end of this book). Compare your actual carbohydrate intake with the target value you calculated. If it is way below the carbohydrate target, you have some serious carb eating to do! If you're within 50 grams, or even a little over, your carbohydrate target, that's fine! Use the carbo-hydrate counter to help you plan a higher carb intake. Remember, this is a rough estimate; you may need a little more or less carbohydrate, depending on how you feel.

Chapter 5

WHICH CARBOHYDRATE FOODS ARE BEST?

*C*arbohydrate foods include breads, breakfast cereals, rice and pasta, fruit and vegetables, especially starchy vegetables such as new potatoes, corn and dried peas and beans. There are smaller amounts of carbohydrate in dairy foods and in processed foods containing sugars. The carbohydrate foods give you a range of nutrients essential for good health. When you're establishing the overall balance of your diet it is important to consume more of the carbohydrate foods that contain a high proportion of nutrients (we call these "nutrient dense") rather than those without additional vitamins and minerals.

Many active people, especially athletes in heavy training who eat large volumes of food, easily meet their daily nutrient requirements. Their carbohydrate needs, however, are sometimes so high, they simply can't manage the volume they need to eat! Liquid meals or carbohydrate supplements can help these athletes with high-energy requirements meet their energy needs in a less "bulky" way.

■

TODAY, THERE'S ANOTHER VITAL CONSIDERATION IN SELECTING CARBOHYDRATE FOODS TO BOOST YOUR SPORTS PERFORMANCE.
IT IS THE GLYCEMIC INDEX OF A FOOD.

■

THE GLYCEMIC INDEX MADE SIMPLE

Carbohydrate foods that break down quickly during digestion have the highest G.I. values. The blood glucose, or sugar, response is fast and high. In other words the glucose in the bloodstream increases rapidly. Conversely, carbohydrates that break down slowly, releasing glucose gradually into the bloodstream, have low G.I. values. An analogy might be the popular fable of the tortoise and the hare. The hare, just like high G.I. foods, speeds away full steam ahead but loses the race to the tortoise with his slow and steady pace. Similarly, slow and steady low G.I. foods produce a smooth blood sugar curve without wild fluctuations.

For most people most of the time, the foods with low G.I. values have advantages over those with high G.I. values. Figure 1 shows the effect of slow and fast carbohydrate on blood sugar levels.

The substance that produces the greatest rise in blood sugar levels is pure glucose itself. All other foods have less effect when fed in equal amounts of

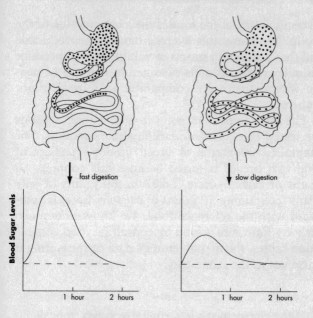

Figure 1. Slow and fast carbohydrate digestion and the consequent levels of sugar in the blood.

carbohydrate. The glycemic index of pure glucose is set at 100, and every other food is ranked on a scale from 0 to 100 according to its actual effect on blood sugar levels.

The glycemic index of a food cannot be predicted from its composition or the glycemic index of related foods. To test the glycemic index, you need real people and real foods. We describe how the glycemic index of a food is measured in the following chapter. There is no easy, inexpensive substitute test. Scientists always follow standardized methods so that results from one group of people can be directly compared with those of another group.

In total, 8 to 10 people need to be tested and the

glycemic index of the food is the average value of the group. We know this average figure is reproducible and that a different group of volunteers will produce a similar result. Results obtained in a group of people with diabetes are comparable to those without diabetes.

The most important point to note is that all foods are tested in equivalent carbohydrate amounts. For example, 100 grams of bread (about 3½ slices of sandwich bread) is tested because this contains 50 grams of carbohydrate. Likewise, 60 grams of jelly beans (containing 50 grams of carbohydrate) is compared with the reference food. We know how much carbohydrate is in a food by consulting food composition tables, the manufacturer's data or measuring it ourselves in the laboratory.

■

THE GLYCEMIC INDEX IS A CLINICALLY PROVEN TOOL IN ITS APPLICATIONS TO DIABETES, APPETITE CONTROL AND REDUCING THE RISK OF HEART DISEASE.

■

HOW CAN I CALCULATE THE GLYCEMIC INDEX OF A MIXED MEAL?

You calculate the glycemic index of a mixed meal by averaging the glycemic index of the different carbohydrate foods in the meal. Let's use hummus on toast as an example: Regular white bread has a glycemic index of 70 and hummus has a glycemic index of 42. If equal amounts of carbohydrate come from the hummus and the bread then you add the G.I. values and divide by two, e.g. $(70 + 42)/2 = 56$.

Let's say the meal contained one-quarter of the carbohydrate from hummus to three-quarters of the carbohydrate from bread; then 25 percent of the glycemic index for hummus would be added to 75 percent of the glycemic index for bread. The following calculation shows how to calculate this.

$$42 \times .25 = 10.5$$
$$70 \times .75 = 52.5$$
$$\text{G.I.} = 10.5 + 52.5 = 63$$

But you really don't need to do calculations. All you need to remember is:

■

LOW G.I. + HIGH G.I. = INTERMEDIATE G.I.

■

Chapter 6

THE GLYCEMIC INDEX: SOME BACKGROUND

HOW THE MILLS CHANGED EVERYTHING

HOW THE GLYCEMIC INDEX CAME TO BE

EARLY CRITICISM

MEASURING THE GLYCEMIC INDEX

For the past 10,000 years, our ancestors survived on a high carbohydrate and low fat diet. They ate their carbohydrates in the form of beans, vegetables and whole cereal grains, and got their sugars from fibrous fruits and berries. Food preparation was a simple process: They ground food between stones and cooked it over the heat of an open fire. The result? All of their food was digested and absorbed slowly, which raised their blood sugar levels more slowly and over a longer period of time.

This diet was ideal for their bodies because it provided slow release energy that helped to delay hunger pangs and provided fuel for working muscles long after the meal was eaten. The slow rise in blood sugar was also kind to the pancreas, the organ that produces insulin.

HOW THE MILLS CHANGED EVERYTHING

As time passed, flours were ground more and more finely and bran was separated completely from the white flour. With the advent of high-speed roller mills in the nineteenth century, it was possible to produce white flour so fine that it resembled talcum powder in appearance and texture. These fine white flours have always been highly prized because they make soft bread and light, airy sponge cakes. As incomes grew, people pushed their peas and beans aside and started eating more meat. As a consequence, the composition of the average diet changed, in that we began to eat more fat and because the type of carbohydrate in our diet changed, it became more quickly digested and absorbed. Something we didn't expect happened, too: The blood sugar rise after a meal was higher and more prolonged, stimulating the pancreas to produce more insulin.

THE PANCREAS PRODUCES INSULIN

The pancreas is a vital organ near the stomach, and its main job is to produce the hormone insulin. Carbohydrate stimulates the secretion of insulin more than any other component of food. The slow absorption of the carbohydrate in our food means that the pancreas doesn't have to work so hard and needs to produce less insulin. If the pancreas is overstimulated over a long period of time, it may become "exhausted" and type 2 diabetes can develop in genetically susceptible people. Even without diabetes, high insulin levels are undesirable because they increase the risk of heart disease.

Unfortunately, over time, we have begun to eat more "refined" foods and fewer "whole" foods. This new way of eating has brought with it higher blood sugar levels after a meal and higher insulin responses, as well. Though our bodies do need insulin for carbohydrate metabolism, high levels of the hormone have a profound effect on the development of many diseases. In fact, medical experts now believe that high insulin levels are one of the key factors responsible for heart disease and hypertension. Insulin influences the way we metabolize foods, determining whether we burn fat or carbohydrate to meet our energy needs and ultimately determining whether we store fat in our bodies.

MEASURING THE GLYCEMIC INDEX

Scientists use just six steps to determine the glycemic index of a food. Simple as this may sound, it's actually quite a time-consuming process. Here's how it works.

1. An amount of food containing 50 grams of carbohydrate is given to a volunteer to eat. For example, to test boiled spaghetti, the volunteer would be given 200 grams of spaghetti, which supplies 50 grams of carbohydrate (we work this out from food composition tables)—50 grams of carbohydrate is equivalent to 3 tablespoons of pure glucose powder.

2. Over the next two hours (or three hours if the volunteer has diabetes), we take a sample of their blood every 15 minutes during the first hour and thereafter every 30 minutes. The blood sugar level of these blood samples is measured in the laboratory and recorded.

3. The blood sugar level is plotted on a graph and the area under the curve is calculated using a computer program (Figure 2).

4. The volunteer's response to spaghetti (or whatever food is being tested) is compared with his or her blood sugar response to 50 grams of pure glucose (the reference food).

5. The reference food is tested on two or three separate occasions and an average value is calculated. This is done to reduce the effect of day-to-day variation in blood sugar responses.

6. The average glycemic index found in 8 to 10 people is the glycemic index of that food.

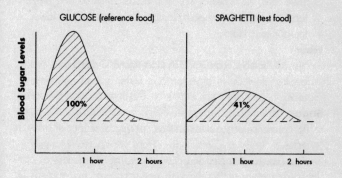

Figure 2. Measuring the glycemic index of a food. The effect of a food on blood sugar levels is calculated using the area under the curve (shaded area). The area under the curve after consumption of the test food is compared with the same area after the reference food (usually 50 grams of pure glucose or a 50 gram carbohydrate portion of white bread).

5 KEY FACTORS THAT INFLUENCE THE GLYCEMIC INDEX

Cooking methods

Cooking and processing increases the glycemic index of a food because it increases the amount of gelatinized starch in the food. Corn flakes is one example.

Physical form of the food

An intact fibrous coat, such as that on grains and legumes, acts as a physical barrier and slows down digestion, lowering a food's G.I. value.

Type of starch

There are two types of starch in foods, amylose and amylopectin. The more amylose starch a food contains, the lower the glycemic index.

Fiber

Viscous, soluble fibers, such as those found in rolled oats and apples, slow down digestion and lower a food's glycemic index.

Sugar

The presence of sugar, as well as the type of sugar, will influence a food's glycemic index. Fruits with a low glycemic index, such as apples and oranges, are high in fructose.

THE KEY IS THE RATE OF DIGESTION

Carbohydrate foods that break down quickly during digestion have the highest G.I. values. Conversely, carbohydrates that break down slowly, releasing glucose gradually into the bloodstream, have low G.I. values.

Low G.I.   less than 55

Intermediate G.I.	55 to 70
High G.I.	more than 70

Take some time to browse through the G.I. tables at the back of this book. Some of the G.I. values may surprise you! At first it's hard to believe that sugar-containing foods may have a lower glycemic index than fibrous, starchy foods like potato. But remember, these blood sugar responses have been measured numerous times and the tests have been repeated by different scientists around the world.

■

THE ONLY WAY TO TELL IF A FOOD HAS A HIGH OR LOW GLYCEMIC INDEX IS TO MEASURE IT.

■

TRICKY TWINS

Circle the food in each of the following pairs that you think will have the lower G.I. value.

Rice	Kellogg's Rice Krispies™
Corn	Corn flakes
Baked potatoes	French fries
Toasted muesli	Untoasted muesli
Whole grain bread	Whole wheat bread

Answers: Rice, corn, baked potatoes, toasted muesli, whole grain bread (depending on the brand).

Chapter 7

WHAT'S YOUR
ACTIVITY LEVEL?

---

*T*he amount of carbohydrate you need depends
on your weight and activity level. Below, we
offer step-by-step guidelines to help you calculate *your* needs.

ACTIVITY LEVEL	GRAMS OF CARBOHYDRATE PER KG BODY WEIGHT PER DAY
Light: Walking, light/easy swimming or cycling; low impact /easy beat aerobic dance *Less than 1 hour per day*	4–5

ACTIVITY LEVEL	GRAMS OF CARBOHYDRATE PER KG BODY WEIGHT PER DAY
Light–moderate: Intermediate aerobic dance class; easy jog; non-competitive tennis (3 sets); volleyball *1 hour per day*	5–6
Moderate: One-hour run; serious training for recreational/competition sports such as soccer, basketball, squash *1–2 hours per day*	6–7
Moderate–heavy: Most professional /elite training for competitive sport such as swimming, tennis, football, distance running (except marathons) *2–4 hours per day*	7–8
Heavy: Training for Ironman events; marathon running/swimming; Olympic distance triathlon *More than 4 hours per day*	8–10

- Activity levels refer to the intensity as well as the duration of the activity.
- Time refers to the amount of time you are physically active during training, not the amount of time at training.
- Body weight refers to ideal or healthy body weight.

Here's an example of how the numbers add up for one athlete.

JESSICA'S CARBOHYDRATE NEEDS

Step 1. Weight   128 lbs. (58 kg)

Step 2. Activity   Moderate level (training for
                                  mid-distance fun runs
                                  such as 5 or 10Ks—
                                  recreational level)
                                  Requires 6–7 g of
                                  carbohydrate per kilogram
                                  per day
                                  **Target carbohydrate
                                  level is:**
                                  6 x 58 = 348 g per day to
                                  7 x 58 = 406 g per day
                                  348–406 g per day

Step 3.   Food record

JESSICA'S FOOD RECORD

MEAL	CARBOHYDRATE COUNT (G)
Breakfast	
1 cup of bran flakes	29
½ cup of milk	6
1 slice of white toast with butter	12
4 ozs. no sugar added fruit juice	15

Meal	Carbohydrate count (g)
Snack	
1 medium banana	27
Lunch	
1 cheese and tomato sandwich on white bread	25
6 ozs. light fruit yogurt	16
1 glass water	0
Snack	
Kavli™ All Natural Whole Grain Crispbread, 4 wafers, with peanut butter	16
1 orange	15
Dinner	
1 small piece of steak	0
1 medium potato	34
½ cup of mixed frozen vegetables	12
½ cup low fat ice cream	15
Snack	
4 Nabisco Social Tea biscuits™	13
Total carbohydrate	**220**

Jessica's carbohydrate count is way below target.

To boost Jessica's carbohydrate intake, add:

1 extra piece of toast at breakfast	12
1 cup split pea soup and 1 cup natural applesauce at lunch	70
1 cup cooked rice pilaf with dinner and increase mixed vegetables to 1 cup	57

MEAL	CARBOHYDRATE COUNT (G)
1 bread roll with dinner	30
8 ozs. of milk with evening snack	
Add 1 tablespoon spreadable fruit on Nabisco Social Tea biscuits™	22

Grand total boosted with the extra carbohydrate foods	**381 g**

This is in the middle of the recommended range for Jessica's weight and activity level. Depending on how she feels, she may need to make slight adjustments depending on variations in the intensity and duration of her training program.

Chapter 8

USING THE GLYCEMIC INDEX TO BOOST SPORTS PERFORMANCE

*T*here are several applications of the glycemic index to sports performance. Sometimes it will be best to choose a high G.I. food, while at other times, a low G.I. food may be more beneficial. Choosing one type of food over another all depends on what you want to accomplish.

To date, most work on the glycemic index and sports performance has concentrated on competition eating and recovery. Over the past few years, however, several studies suggest that eating low to moderate G.I. foods *prior* to an event can prolong endurance. In fact, one study showed that time to exhaustion was 59 percent longer after athletes had eaten a low glycemic index meal!

A HIGH CARBOHYDRATE DIET IS ESSENTIAL
FOR PEAK ATHLETIC PERFORMANCE

A high carbohydrate diet is a must for optimum athletic performance because it produces the largest stores of muscle glycogen. As we have previously described, the carbohydrate we eat is stored in the body in the form of glycogen in the muscles and liver. A small amount of carbohydrate (about 1 teaspoon) circulates as glucose in the blood. When you're exercising at a high intensity, your muscles rely on glycogen and glucose for fuel. Although the body can use fat when you're exercising at lower intensities, fat can't provide the fuel fast enough when you are working very hard. The larger your stores of glycogen and glucose, the longer you can go before fatigue sets in.

Unlike the fat stores in the body that can release almost unlimited amounts of fatty acids, the carbohydrate stores are small, and are fully depleted after two or three hours of strenuous exercise. It's also when blood glucose concentrations begin to decline. If you continue to exercise at the same rate, blood glucose may drop to levels that interfere with brain function and cause disorientation and unconsciousness.

MISCONCEPTIONS ABOUT CARBOHYDRATES

Many athletes and coaches have misconceptions about carbohydrates that can affect athletic performance. In the past we were taught that simple carbohydrates (sugars) were digested and absorbed rapidly while complex carbohydrates (starches) were digested slowly. We assumed (completely incorrectly) that simple carbohydrates gave the most rapid rises in blood sugar while complex carbohydrates produced gradual rises. Unfortunately, these assumptions had no factual or scientific basis. Instead, they were based on structural considerations: Smaller molecules, like sugars, were thought to be easier to digest than larger ones, such as starches. Even though incorrect, the logical nature of these assumptions meant that they were rarely ever questioned. Unfortunately, many people still think sugars are the best source of quick energy and that starches are our best source of sustained energy.

HOW CARBOHYDRATES CAN HELP

Scientific research has so far identified three key applications of the glycemic index to enhance performance.

1. A low G.I. pre-event meal may enhance endurance in prolonged exercise.

2. High G.I. foods or fluids during exercise help to maintain blood sugar levels.

3. High G.I. foods in the recovery phase after exercise help to accelerate glycogen replenishment.

Researchers at the University of Sydney in Australia have found that a low G.I. pre-event meal, at least one hour prior to endurance exercise, can delay fatigue by delivering greater amounts of carbohydrate to the muscle late in exercise. Look at it this way: The low G.I. meal will still be digesting while you exercise and providing an additional source of carbohydrate that you had long forgotten about. Slow-release (low G.I.) carbohydrate is thought to be particularly useful for exercise of long duration when glycogen stores become limited. This is especially true when the ability to consume carbohydrate during the event is difficult or limited. Low G.I. foods, because they are absorbed much more slowly, can be likened to a continuous injection of glucose during the event. This glucose "infusion" can boost energy when fatigue begins to set in.

EAT TO COMPETE: CARBOHYDRATE LOADING

Carbohydrate (or glycogen) loading increases the body's store of glycogen in the liver and muscles. The extra glycogen provides additional fuel for endurance exercise when a normal glycogen store won't be sufficient to maintain stamina.

To carbohydrate load, athletes used to go through a glycogen depletion phase that made the muscles "hungry" for glycogen. These early regimes were like torture, because athletes felt tired and irritable. This way of eating also made it difficult for athletes to maintain their motivation and concentration. After two or three days of the depletion phase, the athletes would then eat a high carbohydrate diet, providing 9 to 10 g of carbohydrate for every kilogram of body weight, for another three days. During this time glycogen stores increased by 200 or 300 percent.

In recent times, athletes have been using a modified carbohydrate loading regimen that results in a similar glycogen store without the unpleasant "depletion" phase. Athletes simply taper training during the week prior to competition and consume a high carbohydrate diet as described above for two to three days prior to competition.

Do you need to carbohydrate load?

All athletes need an adequate normal store of carbohydrate to maximize performance. Carbohydrate loading, in its true sense, is only needed for endurance athletes exercising for longer than two hours, such as those people competing in triathlons, marathons, centuries or other endurance events.

What about the glycemic index and carbohydrate loading?

At present there is insufficient scientific evidence to recommend a particular glycemic index for carbohydrate loading. It appears that high G.I. diets may result in higher muscle glycogen levels in non-athletes. It would seem reasonable to propose that a higher G.I. diet may facilitate more effective glycogen loading, but further research is needed.

■

CARBOHYDRATE LOADING INCREASES
THE BODY'S STORE OF GLYCOGEN,
WHICH HELPS TO PREVENT FATIGUE
DURING ENDURANCE EVENTS.

■

Chapter 9

THE PRE-COMPETITION MEAL

S ince the pre-competition meal has the potential to either make or break your performance on event day, what you eat should not be left to chance. Work on a dietary strategy using the following guidelines, then practice these principles before a training session to allow yourself time to fine tune your pre-competition meal.

GUIDELINES

- Eat two to four hours before the event. This allows time for your pre-competition meal to empty from the stomach. Allow four hours for a larger meal.

- Make the meal high in carbohydrate for maximum energy.
- Fill up, but don't overeat. Eat a comfortable amount of food.
- Keep your fat intake down for this meal, because fat slows digestion.
- Go for a moderate amount of protein. Fill up on carbohydrates instead.
- Aim for a moderate amount of fiber. Too much high fiber food could cause bloating, diarrhea and discomfort during the competition.
- Drink your meal. If you're too nervous, or you feel it's too early in the morning to eat, try a sports drink or liquid meal (such as Ensure Light or Super Shake) so that you can maintain your energy with liquid food.
- Practice. Experiment with different meals to find out what works best for you.

READY?

On your mark

Remember, the pre-event meal won't work miracles if your training diet is inadequate. Make sure you are eating well generally, especially for the week leading up to competition.

Get set

Use these pre-competition guidelines to help you plan your pre-event meal.

Go!

During exercise, replace fluids and carbohydrates regularly as you go.

THE PRE-EVENT MEAL

Athletes like to eat foods that won't be too heavy or fibrous. If you want to try low G.I. options, choose foods that are not too fibrous or gas producing—taking a bathroom break during exercise can be very inconvenient! Suitable light and low G.I. foods include pasta, some varieties of rice (Basmati, brown, Uncle Ben's Converted), low G.I. breads (those with barley or whole grains) and some breakfast cereals (such as old-fashioned oats). For examples of low G.I. meal foods, see the table on page 45.

TWO QUICK ANSWERS

How much should I eat before the event?

About 1 to 2 grams of carbohydrate for each 2.2 lbs. of body weight (example: 50 to 100 grams of carbohydrate if you weigh 110 lbs., or 75 to 150 grams of carbohydrate if you weigh 165 lbs.)

How soon before?

One to two hours before the event is a good starting point. You should experiment to determine the timing that works best for you.

The following table shows the serving sizes of low G.I. foods containing 50 grams or 75 grams of carbohydrate. (You can adjust the food amounts on the following list to make sure you're taking in the right amount of carbohydrate.) Keep in mind that you won't win any contests if your pre-event meal is jiggling around in your stomach (this will affect a runner more than a cyclist). So test the timing and amount of low G.I. food during your training sessions. Then you'll be ready for the big day. Just don't try it out for the first time on the day of the competition!

SERVING SIZES OF LOW G.I. FOODS TO EAT 1 TO 2 HOURS BEFORE THE EVENT

Food	Glycemic Index	Serving size = 50 g carbohydrate	Serving size = 75 g carbohydrate
Heavy grain breads, such as pumpernickel	51	3 slices (approx. 3 ozs.)	4 to 5 slices (approx. 5 ozs.)
Spaghetti, cooked	37	1½ cups (6 ozs.)	2¼ cups (10 ozs.)
Oatmeal, cooked	49	2½ cups (20 ozs.)	3½ cups (32 ozs.)
Baked beans	48	medium can (16 ozs.)	1½ medium cans (24 ozs.)
Fruit salad	approx. 50	2½ cups (approx. 16 ozs.)	4 cups (28 ozs.)
Yogurt (low fat)	33	2 containers (16 ozs.)	3 containers (24 ozs.)
Apples	38	3 small or medium (16 ozs.)	4 small (20 ozs.)
Oranges	44	5 small (20 ozs.)	7 small (32 ozs.)
Dried apricots	31	¾ cup (4 ozs.)	1⅓ cups (4 ozs.)

Females who weigh about 110 lbs. should aim to eat 50 to 100 grams of carbohydrate.

Males who weigh about 165 lbs. should aim to eat 75 to 150 grams of carbohydrate.

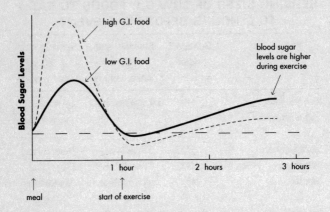

Figure 3. Comparison of the effect of low and high G.I. foods on blood sugar levels during prolonged strenuous exercise. When a pre-event meal of lentils (low glycemic index) was compared with potatoes (high glycemic index), cyclists were able to continue cycling at a high intensity (65 percent of their peak aerobic capacity) for 20 minutes longer after eating the lentil meal. Their blood sugar and insulin levels were significantly higher at the end of exercise, which indicated that the athletes were still absorbing carbohydrate from the small intestine even after 90 minutes of strenuous exercise.

Chapter 10

DURING AN EVENT

---

*H*igh G.I. carbohydrate is the best choice to optimize performance, since the carbohydrate needs to be rapidly available to the muscle as a fuel source. Consuming carbohydrate "on the run" has been shown to delay fatigue because it provides energy to working muscles when the body's own stores of glycogen are low. This is especially true when exercise is prolonged and even glycogen loading cannot prepare the body for the carbohydrate needed to get through the long endurance event.

If you don't have sufficient carbohydrate in your training diet, supplementing carbohydrate during exercise helps you keep pace when your glycogen stores are low. Just remember: This isn't a quick fix to avoid a high carbohydrate training diet! The body needs to obtain most of the carbs from glycogen stored in the muscle during exercise. Outside carbs are a great backup, but it's essential to prepare your body by eating a high-carb training diet each day.

The table below lists high G.I. carbohydrates that are popular during exercise. Athletes usually tolerate sports electrolyte replacement drinks better because they empty from the stomach more quickly.

HIGH G.I. CHOICES SUITABLE DURING EXERCISE

Food	G.I.	Serving Size	Carbohydrate (g)
Gatorade™	78	1 quart	56
Crispbread with honey	73	6 crackers with 1 tablespoon honey	46
Breakfast bar, fruit flavor (such as Kellogg's Nutri-Grain cherry)	78	1 bar	27
Jelly beans	80	24 large (2½ ozs.)	60
Rice cakes	82	7 cakes	50
Honey graham crackers	74	9 squares	50

■

PROLONG YOUR ENDURANCE BY FILLING UP ON FLUIDS AND CARBOHYDRATE REGULARLY THROUGHOUT EXERCISE.

■

Sports or electrolyte replacement drinks are ideal because they encourage greater fluid consumption than water, enhance intestinal absorption of fluid and provide carbohydrate while rehydrating your body all at the same time. They are also less likely to cause gastrointestinal distress than solid foods.

The choice of solid or liquid carbohydrate during exercise is ultimately up to you. But with the current sports/electrolyte formulations providing an optimal quickly absorbed source of carbohydrates, it is hard to look past this as a primary option. Many athletes choose a combination of sports drinks and comfortable solid foods they have tried while in training. During prolonged exercise, solid foods fill up that empty feeling in your stomach.

■

USE THIS BOOK AS A GUIDE TO START EXPERIMENTING WITH DIFFERENT FOODS AND FLUIDS THROUGHOUT TRAINING SESSIONS. DISCOVER FOR YOURSELF WHAT FEELS MOST COMFORTABLE AND WORKS BEST FOR YOU.

■

Many of the popular foods used during exercise over the years were adopted because they were convenient or easy to eat, rather than because they had a high glycemic index. The ever popular banana, for example, has an intermediate G.I. value. Eating a banana during exercise isn't wrong, but when the pace is really on and you want a fast energy supply, a more rapidly absorbing high G.I. option would be better. In prolonged exercise, you should aim to consume 30 to 60 g of carbohydrate per hour over the session or event.

During long events, a combination of comfortable foods (whatever their glycemic index), along with the high G.I. options, will provide the best variety and feelings of psychological well being. The occasional mini chocolate bar may not be the best high G.I. fuel during exercise from a scientific point of view, but in the final stages of the Ironman, it may boost your morale enough to keep you going. These psychological factors cannot be underestimated.

Chapter 11

RECOVERY: THE CASE FOR HIGH G.I. FOODS

*A*fter exercise, your muscles are hungry for carbohydrate. If you postpone consuming carbohydrate after exercise, you'll delay muscle glycogen replenishment and could become fatigued.

- If you're a recreational exerciser, an adequate carbohydrate intake over the next few days will ensure that your muscles are ready for another session.
- If you're participating in strenuous training, particularly when two or more training sessions are part of your daily routine, rapid glycogen replenishment is vital. Eat or drink carbohydrate within 30 minutes of strenuous exercise when you plan to train again within a few

hours. On consecutive days of competition, this recovery strategy will also assist in restocking your glycogen stores for the next event.

RECOVERY AFTER EXERCISE

In the immediate post exercise period, high G.I. carbohydrates are best because they are digested and absorbed much faster and stimulate more insulin—the hormone responsible for getting glucose into the muscle and storing it as glycogen. Most athletes prefer high carbohydrate drinks because they are usually thirsty rather than hungry after strenuous exercise. A drink also aids rehydration.

Sports or electrolyte replacement drinks are ideal for replacing fluids and providing an immediate and convenient source of high G.I. carbohydrate.

After this initial "dose" of recovery carbs, try to make sure your next meal or snack (within two hours) includes intermediate to high G.I. foods.

RECOVERY FORMULA

The amount of carbohydrate required to kick off the recovery process is about 1.5 grams per kilogram of body weight. Most people need between 75 and approximately 100 grams of carbohydrate in the immediate post exercise period. The table on page 53 outlines a list of convenient high G.I. foods and sports drinks suitable for recovery.

■

POSTPONING CARBOHYDRATE CONSUMPTION
AFTER EXERCISE DELAYS MUSCLE GLYCOGEN
REPLENISHMENT AND CAN CAUSE FATIGUE.

■

SERVING SIZES OF HIGH G.I. FOODS TO ENHANCE RECOVERY

Food	G.I.	Serving size = 75 grams carbohydrate	Serving size = 100 grams carbohydrate
White or brown bread	70	4–5 slices (5 ozs.)	6 slices (6 ozs.)
Kellogg's Rice Krispies™	89	3½ cups (3 ozs. + 8 ozs. milk)	4½ cups (4 ozs. + 12 ozs. milk)
Kellogg's Corn Flakes™	84	2¼ cups (2¼ ozs. + 8 ozs. milk)	3 cups (3 ozs. + 12 ozs. milk)
Watermelon	72	6½ cups (2 lbs.)	8⅔ cups (2½ lbs.)
Honey graham crackers	79	13 squares (3½ ozs.)	18 squares (4½ ozs.)
Rice cakes	82	10 rice cakes (3 ozs.)	14 rice cakes (5 ozs.)
English muffins, toasted	70	3 whole muffins (6 ozs.)	4 whole muffins (8 ozs.)
Instant rice, cooked	87	2 cups (11 ozs.)	2⅔ cups (14 ozs.)
Jelly beans	80	30 large (3 ozs.)	40 large (4 ozs.)
Gatorade™	78	5⅓ cups (42 ozs.)	7 cups (56 ozs.)

Females weighing about 110 lbs. should aim to eat 75 grams of carbohydrate.

Males weighing about 165 lbs. should aim to eat 112 grams of carbohydrate.

■

BETTER FUELING—NOT MORE TRAINING —CAN GIVE YOU THE COMPETITIVE EDGE!

■

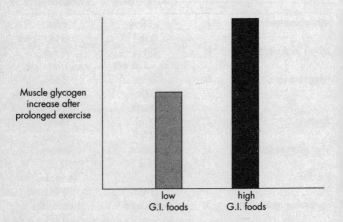

Muscle glycogen increase after prolonged exercise

low G.I. foods   high G.I. foods

Figure 4. Comparison of the effect of low and high G.I. foods on replenishment of muscle glycogen levels after exercise.

Chapter 12

THE IMPORTANCE OF WEIGHT CONTROL

A high carbohydrate, low G.I. diet can help you manage your weight and body fat levels with greater ease. Low G.I. foods help you fill up more easily, which is useful if you need to control your food intake to stay lean or make a weight for competition.

The good news is that carbohydrate foods are *filling*, not *fattening*. Fatty foods, in particular, have only a weak effect on satisfying our appetites relative to the number of calories they provide. Carbohydrate foods make you feel fuller than fats and don't end up on your body in places where you least want them!

HERE'S THE PROOF!

In studies at the University of Sydney in Australia, people were given a range of foods that contained equal numbers of calories, and then their satiety (feeling of fullness and satisfaction after eating) responses were compared. High carbohydrate, low G.I. foods were the most filling and satisfying.

If you need to increase your food intake to gain lean body mass, excessive amounts of low G.I. food may be just too filling. In this case, you need to balance the glycemic index in your meals so you can consume enough food.

■

LOW FAT, LOW G.I. CARBOHYDRATE FOODS HELP YOU TO FEEL FULL AND MORE SATISFIED AFTER EATING.

■

By eating a high carbohydrate diet you will tend to automatically lower your fat intake and, by choosing your carbohydrate from low G.I. foods, make meals and snacks even more satisfying.

EAT MORE, WEIGH LESS

Even when the caloric intake is the same, people eating low G.I. foods may lose more weight than those eating high G.I. foods. In a study in South Africa, the investigators divided overweight women into two groups: One group ate a low calorie, high G.I. diet

and the other, a low calorie, low G.I. diet. The
amount of calories, fat, protein, carbohydrate and
fiber in the diet was the same for both groups—only
the G.I. values of the diets was different. The low G.I.
group included foods such as lentils, pasta, oatmeal
and corn in their diet and excluded high G.I. foods,
including white bread. After 12 weeks, the volunteers
in the group eating low G.I. foods had lost, on average, 20 pounds—4½ pounds more than people in the
group eating the diet of high G.I. foods.

The most significant finding? The two diets affect-
ed blood levels of insulin completely differently. Low
G.I. foods resulted in lower levels of insulin circulat-
ing in the bloodstream. Insulin, you'll remember, is a
hormone that is not only involved in regulating blood
sugar levels, but also plays a key part in when and
how we store fat. High insulin levels often exist in
obese people, in those with high blood fat levels
(either cholesterol or triglyceride) and in those with
heart disease. This study suggested that the low
insulin responses associated with low G.I. foods
helped the body to burn more fat rather than store it.

■

THE REAL AIM IN LOSING WEIGHT IS LOSING BODY FAT.
PERHAPS IT WOULD BE BETTER DESCRIBED AS "RELEAS-
ING" BODY FAT. AFTER ALL, TO LOSE SOMETHING SUG-
GESTS THAT YOU HOPE TO FIND IT AGAIN SOME DAY!

■

If you are still fearful of gaining weight by eating
more pasta, bread and potatoes, consider this: The
body actually has to use up calories to convert the carbohydrate we eat into body fat. The cost is 23 percent

of the available calories—that is, nearly one-quarter of the calories of the carbohydrate are used up just storing it. Naturally, the body is not keen on wasting energy this way. In fact, the body converts carbohydrate to fat only under very unusual situations such as forced overfeeding. The human body prefers the easy option, which is to burn those calories, and it is far more willing to add to our fat stores with the fat that we eat. Conversion of fat in food to body fat is an extremely efficient process and body fat stores are virtually limitless.

FACTORS THAT INFLUENCE BODY WEIGHT

Like most health conditions, there are many different causes for overweight, some of which include our genetic makeup, hormone levels, environmental factors, psychological issues and metabolic considerations.

For most of us, even without much conscious effort, our bodies maintain a relatively constant weight, often despite huge variations in how much we eat. For a proportion of people who are overweight, this apparent balancing of energy intake and output seems lost or inoperative. So, despite every fad diet, every exercise program, even operations and medications, body weight can steadily increase over the years, regardless of all apparent efforts to control it.

It has always been said that our weight is a result of how much we consume in relation to how much we burn up. So, if we take in too much (overeat) and don't burn up enough (don't exercise) we are likely to put on weight.

The question is: how much, of what, is too much?

The answer is not a simple one: Not all foods that we eat are equal and no two bodies are the same, given the wide variety of special factors we've outlined above.

WHAT'S INVOLVED?

As we mentioned earlier, people are overweight for many different reasons. Some people believe they gain weight just from looking at food, while others say they have only to walk past a bakery to pack on a few extra pounds. Still other folks blame themselves because they eat too much. It is clear that a combination of social, genetic, dietary, metabolic, psychological (and emotional) factors combine to influence our weight.

YOUR FAMILY TREE

Research shows us that a child born to overweight parents is much more likely to be overweight than one whose parents were not overweight. It may sound like an excuse, but studies in twins provide evidence that our body weight and shape are at least partially determined by our genes.

Identical twins tend to be similar in body weight even if they are raised apart. Even twins adopted as infants show the body-fat profile of their true parents rather than that of their adoptive parents. These findings suggest that our genes are a stronger determinant of weight than our environment, which includes the food we eat.

How do genes play a role? It seems that information

stored in our genes governs our tendency to store calories as either fat or as lean muscle tissue. Overfeeding
a large group of identical twins confirmed that within
each pair, weight gain was similar. The amount of
weight gained between sets of identical twins varied
greatly, however. From this, researchers concluded that
our genes control the way our bodies respond to
overeating. Some sets of twins gained a lot of weight,
while others gained only a little, even though all were
consuming an equivalent amount of excess calories.

IT'S NOT JUST GENETICS

Despite a genetic predisposition, you can only gain weight if
you take in more energy than you use. We know that obesity
has many causes—for example, eating too much, exercising
too little, genetics, aging, eating a high fat diet—all play a
part. But what it all boils down to is that if we take in too much
(overeat) and don't burn up enough (don't exercise) we are
likely to put on weight.

All this isn't to say that if your parents were
overweight, you should resign yourself to being overweight. But it may help you understand why you have
to watch your weight while other people seemingly
don't have to watch theirs.

So, if you were born with a tendency to be overweight, why does it matter what you eat? The answer
is that foods (or more correctly, nutrients) are not
equal in their effects on body weight. In particular,
the way the body responds to dietary fat makes mat-
ters worse.

Some scientists believe that fat is fattening because

the body has a very limited ability to store protein and carbohydrate but a very *large* capacity to store fat. Our bodies burn protein and carbohydrate first, and preferentially store dietary fat. Every day we will burn virtually all the carbohydrate and protein we ingest. In a steady state of weight balance, though, the amount of fat we burn each day must equal the amount we eat. (If we eat a high-fat diet, then our body fat stores must expand so that the level of free fatty acids in the blood is high enough to correspond to what we're eating. That's why a high fat diet brings about a high fat body.)

COUNTING THE CALORIES IN OUR NUTRIENTS

All foods contain calories. Often the caloric content of a food is considered a measure of how fattening it is. Of all the nutrients in food that we consume, carbohydrate yields the fewest calories per gram.

carbohydrate	4 calories per gram
protein	4 calories per gram
alcohol	7 calories per gram
fat	9 calories per gram

While you may not have been born owning the best set of genes for the current environment, you can still influence your weight by the lifestyle choices you make. The message is simply this: If you believe that you are at risk of being overweight, you should think seriously about minimizing fat and eating more carbohydrate.

HOW FAST YOUR MOTOR RUNS

Our genetic makeup also underlies our metabolism, which is basically how many calories we burn per minute. Bodies, like cars, differ in this regard. A V-8 consumes more fuel to run than a small four-cylinder car. A bigger body usually requires more calories than a smaller one.

Everyone has a resting metabolic rate, which is a measure of the amount of calories our bodies use when we are at rest. When a car is stationary, the engine idles—using just enough fuel to keep the motor running. When we are asleep, our engine keeps running, too (for example, our heart keeps beating) and we use a minimum number of calories. This is our basal metabolic rate.

When we start exercising, or even just moving around, the number of calories, or the amount of fuel we use, increases. However, the largest amount (around 70 percent) of the calories used in a 24-hour period, are those used to maintain our basic body functioning.

Since our resting metabolic rate is where most of the calories we eat are used, it is a significant determinant of our body weight. The lower your resting energy expenditure, the greater your risk of gaining weight, and vice versa.

Chapter 13

CASE STUDY #1: JIM

Jim is an 18-year-old college football player who recently moved from a small, rural town to join one of the best college teams in the country. Playing college (and eventually professional) football was Jim's dream. Wanting to make a big impression during his first few weeks at training, Jim gave his all. At first he felt fine, but after one week of training twice almost every day he felt exhausted, and was frankly "off the pace." Sensing that Jim was struggling, the coach took him aside and recommended he speak to a registered dietitian about his diet and recovery strategies.

JIM'S WEEKLY TRAINING PROGRAM

Morning weight/circuit training: 2 or 3 sessions per week of 1 to 1½ hours

Afternoon football/fitness sessions: 4 sessions of 2 to 2½ hours per week

---

CONSULTATION WITH THE SPORTS DIETITIAN

Jim was a bit wary about changing his diet; he wondered how eating differently could help him on the football field. The dietitian explained that carbohydrates were the key to energy and recovery. His diet at the moment was far too low in carbohydrate to get him through the tough pre-season training. The dietitian also explained that eating carbohydrate regularly was important, and fueling up immediately (within 30 minutes) after training sessions helped to replace the body's carbohydrate stores more quickly. Timing was important because between morning and afternoon training his body had less than six hours to refuel. More rapidly absorbing carbs or those with an intermediate to high G.I. values were also better for refueling as they replenished the body's carbohydrate or glycogen levels faster.

The dietitian also explained that to help Jim maintain his body weight and stay lean he should:

- use lean meats or cut off the fat
- remove skin from chicken
- use reduced-fat dairy products
- minimize use of oils, butter or margarine

HIGH G.I. FUEL TO THE RESCUE

Jim noticed the other players were already using foods and sports drinks to their advantage. They consumed sports drinks with glucose (high glycemic index) to begin the refueling and rehydration process right after training and chose intermediate to high G.I. breads, cereals or fruit to boost their recovery (French bread, Cheerios, Corn Chex, granola bars, pineapple or watermelon). These foods were available at training so he could start the refueling process before traveling home.

The dietitian also organized cooking classes to give him the confidence to prepare different carbohydrate-based meals for himself. But Jim now knew that when recovery time was short, higher G.I. carbohydrates were best.

RESULTS

Jim noticed the difference in his performance after being on the high carbohydrate diet for only a few days. He felt fresher at afternoon training and could really power through the sprint sessions, which had been like torture before. Including more carbohydrate in his diet and refueling with higher G.I. carbohydrates really helped him. He knew he still had a lot of work to do before the competition season kicked off, but with the right fuel, a great attitude and some raw talent he knew he was ready for some of his best ever performances.

MEAL PLAN FOR JIM

Aim: To provide sufficient carbohydrate and energy and to assist recovery rate by incorporating high G.I. liquids and intermediate to high G.I. meals after training.

NOTES ON G.I.

8:30 A.M. Immediately post training

1 quart sports/electrolyte drink (Gatorade™)

POST TRAINING

9:00 A.M. Breakfast

Intermediate to high G.I. choices

1 piece of fruit	Pineapple, watermelon
2 cups of cereal	Puffed wheat, corn flakes, raisin bran
2 cups of 2% milk	
2 slices white or whole wheat toast (no butter) with 1 tablespoon honey	White or whole wheat kaiser roll or French bread
1 glass of fruit juice (8 ozs.)	Pineapple

11:30 A.M. Snack

1 sandwich with 3 ozs. lean meat filling (turkey breast, lean roast beef)
1 piece of fruit (any type)
1 nonfat yogurt (8 ozs.)

1:00 P.M. Lunch

3 slices rye bread filled with 3 ozs. boiled ham and 2 ozs. American cheese or any of the following: lean meat, chicken, reduced fat cheese, egg, canned tuna in spring water or canned salmon
2 pieces of fresh fruit (any type)

1 pint (16 ozs.) of low fat, flavored milk

2:30 P.M. Snack

Intermediate to high G.I. choices

Fruit smoothie or a liquid meal
(such as Ensure Light or Super Shake)

3:30–5:30 P.M. Pre- and during training

2 quarts of sports/electrolyte drink

High G.I. drink Gatorade™ (78)

5:30 P.M. After training

1 quart sports/electrolyte drink or
   carb loader

High G.I. drink for recovery

7:00 P.M. Dinner

Serving lean meat (5 ozs.),
   or skinless chicken (6 ozs.), or
   fish (8 ozs.)—grilled or cooked
   with minimum oil

Large serving of rice (1⅓ cups),
   or pasta (3 cups) or 2 medium
   potatoes

High G.I. rice on training
nights, pasta most others

1 cup serving of vegetables or large
   tossed green salad (no-oil dressing)

4 slices of white bread or 2 rolls
   (no butter)

High G.I. French bread
on training nights

9:00 P.M. Snack

2 pieces of fresh fruit in a smoothie
   or fruit and yogurt

DIETARY ANALYSIS:

ENERGY: 4458 calories	**FAT:** 74 g (15%)
PROTEIN: 189 g (17%)	**CARBOHYDRATE:** 759 g (68%)

Chapter 14

CASE STUDY #2: ANALISE

*A*nalise, a 16-year-old full-time ballet student, had a dream: to be a dancer with a major ballet company. When she started to mature at 13, she found she could no longer eat anything as she used to. Extra weight started to pile on. First she tried all the diets given to her by the other ballet students, but she always felt hungry and craved chocolate. Getting nowhere by herself, her mother took her to see a sports dietitian.

■ ■ ■

CONSULTATION WITH THE SPORTS DIETITIAN

At their first meeting the dietitian took a history of Analise's weight and eating patterns and found that a typical day's meals for Analise included:

- A slice of white toast with butter and a cup of strong black tea for breakfast
- Two crispbreads with butter and a cup of black tea for a morning snack
- A green salad, an apple and a cup of black tea for lunch
- A chocolate bar and a can of diet cola during the afternoon (waiting at the train station)
- Steamed veggies, sometimes steamed chicken and a cup of black tea for dinner
- A chocolate bar or chocolate cookies and tea for an evening snack

The dietitian explained that this diet was high in fat and too low in protein, carbohydrate, calcium and iron. She explained that:

- Gaining a little body weight and fat is part of the maturation process and that the best way to control body fat was with a sensible diet, not starving.
- Cravings are to be expected when you're hungry. After working hard in class all day with virtually no food, chocolate is just too tempting. Eating more carbohydrate on a regular basis would help Analise control her chocolate cravings.
- Analise needed a dietary strategy to give her sufficient fuel to get through the day without feeling hungry. Carbohydrates (especially low G.I. carbs) would help her to feel fuller, give her

more energy and provide less fat than other foods she'd been eating.

Analise's meal plan, based on reducing fat intake and boosting carbohydrate, meant eating more pasta, rice, bread, fruit and vegetables and less high fat food such as butter and chocolate. Chocolate was not totally out of the question, but she had to cut back to get her body fat levels going in the right direction. The dietitian also explained that reducing the cups of tea would help Analise maintain adequate iron levels, because the tannin in tea reduces iron absorption.

Analise had some questions about the meal plan.

Could she really lose weight eating this much?

The dietitian explained that the size or appearance of foods is often deceiving. Although some high fat foods like chocolate look compact, and foods like bread and vegetables may take up more space on the plate, the fat and calorie values of high fat foods are much greater than those of bread and vegetables. The fat figures in the back of this book were a real surprise to Analise. She was also surprised to learn that the fat we eat is converted into body fat faster and easier than anything else we eat.

Should she cut out chocolate all together?

The dietitian explained that giving up chocolate is really not necessary and is almost impossible unless you live somewhere where there's no chocolate at all. Eating chocolate as a treat, not as a substitute meal, is the key.

How could she avoid feeling too full and having a bloated stomach during class?

Foods with a high fiber content (including many salad veggies) produce more gas in the intestine, which can cause bloating. The dietitian showed Analise how she could increase the intake of low G.I. carbs throughout the day without feeling bloated.

RESULTS

At first Analise kept thinking that she was eating too much. But she was able to avoid the chocolate vending machine on the station platform on the way home because she felt fuller during the day. The really high carb, low G.I. foods reduced her hunger. Her body fat level (measured with body fat or skinfold calipers) dropped steadily each week. She thought it almost unbelievable to be able to drop fat without starving! An added bonus was her improved energy levels and concentration in class, not to mention her mood, which was more relaxed and cheerful.

ANALISE'S MEAL PLAN

Aim: To provide a regular supply of carbohydrate, with less fat. The glycemic index should be intermediate to low to assist with satiety.

NOTES ON G.I.	
8:00 A.M. Breakfast	**Intermediate to low G.I.**
1 piece of fruit	Fresh apple, grapefruit, kiwi
½–⅔ cup bran cereal	All Bran™, oats, Raisin Bran™
4 ozs. skim milk	
1 slice whole grain toast (no butter) and 1 teaspoon spreadable fruit	Oat, barley or mixed grain breads
1 cup decaffeinated coffee	

10:30 A.M. Snack

Nonfat fruit yogurt with artificial
  sweetener

1:00 P.M. Lunch

1 sandwich—protein options include: 2 ozs. of chicken, turkey, canned tuna in water, salmon, reduced fat cheese, lean ham or roast meat	Oat, barley or heavy grain bread
2 cups of salad with 2 tablespoons light dressing	
1 piece of fruit	Peach, pear or plum
Water or decaf diet beverage	

3:30 P.M. Snack

1 raisin toast or ½ English muffin with 1 teaspoon jam	Raisin bread or grain muffin

7:00 P.M. Dinner

3 oz. serving of lean meat, or
  4 ozs. skinless chicken or 5 ozs.

7:00 P.M. Dinner

grilled fish, all cooked in minimum
or no oil

1 medium potato or 1 cup pasta or
⅔ cup rice

1 cup serving of vegetables or salad
with 2 tablespoons light dressing

Water or decaf diet beverage

Intermediate to low G.I.

New boiled potatoes, pasta or
Basmati or brown rice

9:30 P.M. Snack

1 8 oz. glass of skim milk

1 slice raisin toast with 1 teaspoon
spreadable fruit

DIETARY ANALYSIS:

ENERGY: 1305 calories
FAT: 20 g (14%)
CALCIUM: 1225 mg (daily
calcium requirement for
16-year-old female is
1200-1500 mg)

PROTEIN: 78 g (24%)
CARBOHYDRATE: 215 g (66%)
IRON: 14–18 mg (above the
recommended daily intake)

Chapter 15

CASE STUDY #3:
IAN

---

*I*an is a 26-year-old physical education teacher and enthusiastic triathlete. He has competed in the Olympic distance for the past five years but is now trying to qualify for the Ironman triathlon in Hawaii. Ian wanted everything to be just right for his first Ironman race so he could qualify. He approached a sports dietitian to help him plan his dietary strategy and brought a list of questions to ask.

HOW MUCH CARBOHYDRATE DOES HE NEED IN HIS TRAINING DIET?

The approximate amount of carbohydrate Ian needs is calculated by multiplying his weight by the carbohydrate requirement appropriate for his activity level.

Ian's weight:	165 lbs. (75 kg)
Approximate carbohydrate requirement for his activity level (see page 32):	8 g/kg
Daily carbohydrate needs for training:	75 x 8 = 600 g

This amount of carbohydrate may be too difficult to achieve with food. Liquid carbohydrate supplements (such as sports drinks) can help boost carbohydrate intake.

IAN'S TRAINING PROGRAM

	A.M. TRAINING	P.M. TRAINING
Monday	1.8-mile swim	Track session + 4-mile run
Tuesday	1.8-mile swim	60-mile cycle
Wednesday	Rest	9-mile run
Thursday	1.8-mile swim	60-mile cycle
Friday	1.8-mile swim	30-mile easy cycle
Saturday	93-mile cycle	1.8-mile swim
Sunday	Rest	18-mile run

Ian's Vital Statistics
Height: 5'8" (70 inches)
Weight: 165 lbs. (has lost 9 lbs. over the past 3 months)
Sum of 8 skinfolds: 50 mm (indicates that Ian is very lean)

HOW CAN HE INCORPORATE THE GLYCEMIC INDEX INTO HIS TRAINING DIET?

Ian can incorporate the glycemic index into his diet mainly by including high G.I. drinks (such as sports drinks) during and after training. Intermediate to high G.I. foods after training also help to speed up recovery. At other times, it's more important to eat sufficient carbohydrate—whatever the glycemic index. Most athletes requiring the amount of carbohydrate that Ian does will feel more comfortable with moderate to lower fiber carbohydrate choices (such as white bread, white rice and pasta instead of the whole grain varieties, for example). Otherwise the sheer volume of the carbohydrate and fiber becomes too bulky and bloating.

WHY HAS HE BEEN SO FATIGUED LATELY?

Fatigue is a generalized symptom that has numerous causes. Dietary factors that should be considered include:

- **Low iron intake.** If your iron levels are low, then increased amounts of high iron foods need to be included in your diet. Iron deficiency occurs even in athletes with adequate iron intake, and is more common in endurance athletes.
- **Inadequate carbohydrate intake.** It's possible to feel fatigued if your muscle glycogen stores are low, which suggests that you're consuming inadequate amounts of carbohydrate throughout the day. Tiredness can also be due to low blood sugar, which can happen if there's a long period between meals. Low blood sugar (hypo-

glycemia) commonly occurs in early morning or afternoon training sessions when you consume insufficient amounts of carbohydrate before the session.

- **Overtraining.** Having too many strenuous workouts is a common problem with endurance athletes. Training programs need to be tailored to the individual, incorporating their personal needs for sleep and taking into account their occupational demands.

- **Viral illness.** A number of medical conditions—not just viruses—are potential causes of fatigue. Ian would benefit from a referral to a sports physician and an exercise physiologist to help determine which factors in particular are causing his fatigue.

DOES HE NEED TO GLYCOGEN LOAD PRIOR TO THE EVENT?

Since the event will be longer than 2 hours (about 11 hours actually), yes! The meal plan outlined below shows how he can glycogen load using the modified regimen. This regimen involves tapered training and a high carbohydrate diet three to four days prior to the race. The diet should provide about 9 to 10 g of carbohydrate per kg of body weight. Check the meal plan for guidance.

WHAT WOULD BE THE BEST PRE-EVENT MEAL?

Ian would benefit from trying a low G.I. meal in practice to see how this worked for him. To maintain gastric comfort, the best low G.I. options would include lower fiber choices such as white pasta, rolled oats, or a liquid low fat meal (Ensure Light or Super Shake, for example).

HOW COULD HE MAINTAIN ENERGY THROUGHOUT THE EVENT?

During the event, maintaining energy and hydration will be a major factor influencing his performance. Sports drinks would be the best option to replace energy and fluids during the race. Because sports drinks have a high G.I. they will be a rapidly absorbed and easily available source of carbohydrate. Other high G.I. options include carbohydrate gels, jelly beans or honey sandwiches on high G.I. (white French) bread. Because Ian will only be able to carry a small amount of the high G.I. food options, the sports drink will probably provide the basis of his refueling strategy with foods offering minor support.

To prevent boredom and boost morale, some of the other offerings at the aid stations (chocolate chip cookies, sandwiches, colas) could be included in smaller quantities as treats. These provide more of a psychological incentive than physiological boost. Although a little caffeine in the cola drink may help with fatigue later in the race due to its stimulant properties, Ian needs to limit caffeine ingestion to avoid dehydration problems (because it takes longer to empty from the stomach, caffeine can compromise hydration). Caffeine may also be subject to drug testing.

IAN'S MEAL PLAN

Aim: To provide sufficient carbohydrate and nutrition for peak performance. The meal plan should include intermediate to high G.I. meals or snacks after training sessions to help maximize the rate of glycogen replacement.

NOTES ON G.I.

Regular training	Post training intermediate to high G.I. choices	Loading phase
Breakfast		
1–2 pieces of fresh fruit	Pineapple, watermelon	Same breakfast
2 cups General Mills Honey Nut Cheerios™ cereal	Kellogg's Rice Krispies™, Quaker Puffed Wheat™, General Mills Total™	
1 cup (8 oz.) 2% milk		
3 slices of toast with 1 tablespoon honey (no butter)	Kaiser roll or French bread	
16 ozs. orange juice		
Snack		
1 banana and 2 oatmeal raisin cookies (2 oz.)		Same as for training plan but add in an additional banana or a low fat fruit muffin
8 oz. glass of juice (any type)		
Lunch		
3 slices rye bread (made with 6 ozs. of cheese, chicken, lean meat, egg, tuna or salmon)		Same lunch but add in ½ jelly sandwich for extra carbohydrate

Regular training	Post training intermediate to high G.I. choices	Loading phase
1 piece fruit 8 ozs. Gatorade™		

Snack

Fruit smoothie made with 8 ozs. 2% milk		Use a liquid meal (such as Ensure Light or Super Shake) or carb loader.

Before and during training:
  Sports drink (volume
  dependent on session
  type and duration)—
  at least 1 quart
		Be sure to replace
		fluids

Dinner

Medium serving of lean
  meat or skinless
  chicken (5 ozs.), or fish
  (6–8 ozs.) or a
  vegetarian meal
		Same dinner

Large serving of
  potato, rice or
  pasta (1½–2 cups)
	High G.I. rice (such
	as cooked instant
	rice); great after
	hard afternoon
	training sessions	

Medium serving of
  vegetables or tossed
  green salad (at least
  1 cup) with fat free
  dressing		

4 slices of bread or two rolls	high G.I. bread (kaiser roll, French bread)	
2 pieces of fresh fruit	Pineapple, watermelon	
1 glass any juice (8 oz.)		

Snack

4 pieces raisin toast with jelly or honey	Add in a carb-loader drink or a liquid meal (such as Ensure Light or Super Shake)

1 glass fruit juice

DIETARY ANALYSIS (TRAINING):	DIETARY ANALYSIS (LOADING):
ENERGY: 4214 calories	ENERGY: 4531 calories
PROTEIN: 168 g (16%)	PROTEIN: 171 g (15%)
FAT: 86 g (18%)	FAT: 88 g (17%)
CARBOHYDRATE: 692 g (66%)	CARBOHYDRATE: 767g (68%)

THE PRE-EVENT MEAL PLAN FOR IAN

This meal should be consumed about two to three hours prior to competition. Ian had tried out the low G.I. meal in training and wanted to use it in competition. The meals he found most comfortable included:

- Liquid meal (Ensure Light or Super Shake) plus a serving of stewed apple G.I. = 39
- Rolled oats with skim milk and orange juice G.I. = 44
- Lentil soup and grapes   G.I. = 47

RESULTS

Ian went on to qualify for Hawaii. Being prepared for this race was crucial to his best performance. Ian described the Hawaii Ironman as "awesome"—one of the best experiences of his life—and it was made more enjoyable by being well prepared and well fueled.

Chapter 16

CASE STUDY #4:
JOHN

---

*J*ohn is a single man who lives at home. He works as a full-time firefighter and takes college courses at night. As an athlete, John competes in bi- and triathlons. He wants to lose 12 pounds, and believes his physical stamina and athletic performance will improve at an optimal weight of 175 pounds.

JOHN'S TRAINING PROGRAM

Runs: 4 to 6 times a week for 40 minutes (3 miles)
Bikes: 3 times a week for 90 minutes
Weight trains: 5 to 7 times a week for 30 minutes

John's Vital Statistics
Age: 25
Height: 5'9"
Weight: 187 pounds (although muscular, John is still at 110 percent of reasonable body weight for height and body frame. He has gained 12 pounds in the past 9 years)
Goal weight: 170 pounds

JOHN'S "BEFORE" DIET:

Breakfast: Two to three cups Rice Chex, 16 ozs. 2% milk
Snack: Banana, pear, 2 carrots
Lunch: Two slices white sandwich bread, 3 ozs. roast beef, 2 ozs. pretzels, 1 cup strawberries, 32 ozs. Gatorade
Dinner: Grilled steak (16 ozs.), 1½ cups green beans with approximately 2 tablespoons butter, 2 cups linguine with approximately 1 cup cream sauce, 32 ozs. Gatorade
Late night snack: Twenty saltines, 32 ozs. Gatorade

JOHN'S "BEFORE" NUTRITIONAL ANALYSIS:

Calories: 5500
Carbohydrate: 554 g (41%)
Protein: 244 g (18%)
Fat: 252 g (41%)
G.I.: 77

CONSULTATION WITH THE DIETITIAN

Even taking his extreme workout schedule into account, John is overconsuming calories by about 50 percent. Even in an athlete's body, this means weight gain (in the form of body fat). All of the macronutrients in his diet (carbohydrates, protein and fat) need to be reduced to bring the calorie level down to a reasonable level. John needs to reduce his caloric intake to 2800 calories, which will meet his basal metabolic requirements as well as his workout energy needs.

G.I.-SPECIFIC COUNSELING:

John is consuming a high G.I. diet. In addition to reducing his caloric intake in the forms of protein foods (steak and roast beef, for example) and his condiments (such as butter and cream sauces), he will also need to reduce his carbohydrates.

By choosing low G.I. cereals (such as Bran Buds, muesli, old-fashioned oatmeal) instead of high G.I. types (including Rice Chex and corn flakes), and low G.I. breads (such as whole wheat pita, 100% whole wheat or whole grain pumpernickel bread) instead of white sandwich bread, he would feel fuller for longer periods of time. His high G.I. snacks could be replaced with light yogurt or low fat milk, oatmeal or Social Tea biscuits and fruit. One 32-ounce bottle of Gatorade during and after a workout period would suffice on a daily basis as long as he consumed at least 80 ounces of water as well.

JOHN'S NEW, LOW G.I. MENU:

Breakfast: Two cups Quaker Oats oat bran cereal, 12 ozs. 1% milk, large apple, water

Snack: One cup grapes

Lunch: Two slices whole grain pumpernickel, 3 ozs. lean roast beef, 1 tablespoon mayonnaise, a sandwich bag of raw vegetables (baby carrots, celery, pepper strips, for example), large pear, 2 oatmeal cookies, water

Snack: Low fat granola bar, 8 ozs. 1% milk

Dinner: One and one-half cups long grain rice, 6 ozs. chicken rosemary, 2 cups steamed broccoli with 2 pats butter and 2 tablespoons slivered almonds, water

Snack: Small apple cinnamon muffin (from mix), 8 ozs. 1% milk

---

JOHN'S "AFTER" NUTRITIONAL ANALYSIS:

Calories: 2800
Carbohydrate: 379 g (54%)
Protein: 150 g (21%)
Fat: 77 g (25%)
G.I.: 46

RESULTS

After just five weeks, John had dropped 7½ pounds, came in 66th out of more than 200 competitors in a biathlon and had shortened his mile by 40 seconds. He reached his goal weight of 170 pounds after 10 weeks. It's been four years since John has been incorporating low G.I. foods into his meal/snack planning.

He is still an elite athlete, and maintains a healthy weight of 171 pounds. John tells us: "I never dreamed I could run so fast or bike so long on half the calories I was used to eating!"

Chapter 17

YOUR QUESTIONS ANSWERED

Will a high protein diet benefit sports performance?

Currently, there is no solid evidence that high protein diets benefit sports performance. The effects of high protein diets have not been adequately tested and published in scientific journals where other scientists are able to scrutinize the study design and results of claims. Some high protein diet authors recommend 30 percent of calories from protein and fat and 40% from carbohydrate. That proportion for carbohydrate is much lower—and that for protein higher—than recommended by virtually all of the scientific literature on sports nutrition.

■ ■ ■

If a person were to eat both protein and carbohydrates during training and before a race, how much of each should they eat?

For most people, a training diet should provide approximately 60 percent of calories from carbohydrate, 15 to 20 percent of calories from protein and the rest from fat. To calculate the amount of carbohydrate that's best for you, turn to "What's Your Activity Level?" in Chapter 7.

An athlete's protein needs generally range between 1.2 and 2 g of protein per kilogram of body weight. Prior to competition, there's no specific need for additional protein. In fact, in most cases athletes require extra *carbohydrate* to ensure that liver glycogen and blood sugar levels are optimal. By the way, scientists no longer recommend the glycogen-loading protocols of years past, which endorsed a low carbohydrate, higher protein diet to enhance loading. For more on this subject, see the box "Eat to Compete: Carbohydrate Loading" on page 40.

What should be the overall glycemic index of an athlete's diet?

Good question! Unfortunately, scientists have yet to answer it. There is evidence that diets with a higher glycemic index increase the glycogen storage in the muscle of sedentary individuals. This may help athletes to store glycogen more effectively on a day to day basis. A high glycemic index has been shown to enhance the rate of recovery of muscle glycogen after exercise. During exercise, a high glycemic index is required to provide a rapidly available fuel source.

I am a recreational jogger; what should be the glycemic index of my overall diet?

If you exercise to lose weight, there may be some

benefit in choosing low G.I. carbohydrates at each meal for their high satiety value. Generally speaking, it's important for recreational joggers to have sufficient carbohydrate in their diet for good health and energy. Since the time to restore glycogen after a workout is likely to be longer than for elite athletes, there is less need to have high G.I. carbohydrates immediately after exercise.

What about eating between heats and trials over the day?

There is insufficient scientific evidence to recommend a particular glycemic index between events at present. However, it makes sense to include carbohydrates that are rapidly absorbed (higher G.I. foods) on a regular basis over the day. Eat little and often. Maintain fluid intake to optimize hydration. During shorter (less than one hour) breaks, drinking rapidly absorbed liquids is probably best. For longer breaks, we recommend eating small low fat, high carb snacks (including rice cakes, soft fruits, honey sandwiches, sports bars and so on).

Is there an easy way to tell if a food has a high or low glycemic index?

No. The only way to tell is to measure the blood sugar response to that food. Generally, foods that break down quickly during digestion have the highest G.I. values. The glycemic index cannot be predicted from the chemical composition of the food or the G.I. value of related foods. Milling and grinding break down the cellular structure of grains and tend to speed up the rate of digestion, which increases the glycemic index. Cooking increases the digestibility of starch, and may also increase the glycemic index. It might seem surprising, but removing the dietary fiber in bread, rice or pasta has little effect on the glycemic index. However, the viscous fiber found in fruits and some grains (such as oats and barley) may account for their lower glycemic index values. In some instances, fat slows the digestion process and lowers the glycemic index.

Chapter 18

HOW TO USE THE G.I. TABLES

he following table is an A to Z listing of the glycemic index of commonly eaten foods in the United States and Canada. Approximately 300 different foods are listed, including some new values for foods tested only recently.

The G.I. value shown next to each food is the average for that food using glucose as the standard (i.e., glucose has a G.I. value of 100, with other foods rated accordingly). The average may represent the mean of 10 studies of that food worldwide or only 2 to 4 studies. In a few instances, American data are different from the rest of the world and we show that data rather than the average. Rice and oatmeal fall into this category.

To check on a food's glycemic index, simply look

for it by name in the alphabetic list. You may also find it under a food type—e.g., fruit, cookies.

Included in the tables is the carbohydrate (CHO) and fat content of a sample serving of the food. This is to help you keep track of the amount of fat and carbohydrate in your diet. The sample serving is not the recommended serving—it is just an example. The glycemic index does not depend on your serving size because it is a ranking of the glycemic effect of foods using carbohydrate-equivalent portion sizes. You can eat more of a low G.I. food or less of a high G.I. food and achieve the same blood sugar levels.

Remember when you are choosing foods, the glycemic index isn't the only thing to consider. In terms of your blood sugar levels you should also consider the amount of carbohydrate you are eating. For your overall health the fat, fiber and micronutrient content of your diet is also important. A dietitian can guide you further with good food choices; see "For More Information" on page 108 for advice on finding a dietitian.

■

FOR A SMALL EATER (1,500 CALORIES A DAY),
AIM FOR LESS THAN 50 G FAT A DAY
AND 188 G CARBOHYDRATE.

■

FOR A BIGGER EATER (2,500 CALORIES A DAY),
AIM FOR LESS THAN 80 G FAT A DAY
AND 313 G CARBOHYDRATE.

■

Chapter 19

THE GLYCEMIC INDEX TABLE

A–Z OF FOODS WITH GLYCEMIC INDEX, CARBOHYDRATE & FAT

Food	Glycemic Index	Fat (G per svg.)	CHO (G per svg.)
Agave nectar (90% fructose syrup), 1 tablespoon	11	0	16
All-Bran with extra fiber™, Kellogg's, breakfast cereal, ½ cup, 1 oz.	51 (av)	1	22
Angel food cake, ½ cake, 1 oz.	67	trace	17
Apple, 1 medium, 5 ozs.	38 (av)	0	18
Apple, dried, 1 oz.	29	0	24
Apple juice, unsweetened, 1 cup, 8 ozs.	40	0	29
Apple cinnamon muffin, from mix, 1 muffin	44	5	26
Apricots, fresh, 3 medium, 3 ozs.	57	0	12
canned, light syrup, 3 halves	64	0	14
dried, 5 halves	31	0	13
Apricot jam, no added sugar, 1 tablespoon	55	0	17
Apricot and honey muffin, low fat, from mix, 1 muffin	60	4	27
Bagel, 1 small, plain, 2.3 ozs.	72	1	38
Baked beans, ½ cup, 4 ozs.	48 (av)	1	24
Banana bread, 1 slice, 3 ozs.	47	7	46
Banana, raw, 1 medium, 5 ozs.	55 (av)	0	32
Banana, oat and honey muffin, low fat from mix, 1 muffin	65	4	27
Barley, pearled, boiled, ½ cup, 2.6 ozs.	25 (av)	0	22
Basmati white rice, boiled, 1 cup, 6 ozs.	58	0	50
Beets, canned, drained, ½ cup, 3 ozs.	64	0	5
Black bean soup, ½ cup, 4 ½ ozs.	64	2	19
Black beans, boiled, ¾ cup, 4.3 ozs.	30	1	31
Black bread, dark rye, 1 slice, 1.7 ozs.	76	1	18
Blackeyed peas, canned, ½ cup, 4 ozs.	42	1	16
Blueberry muffin, 1 muffin, 2 ozs.	59	4	27
Bran			
All-Bran with extra fiber™, Kellogg's, ½ cup, 1 oz.	51	1	20

Food	Glycemic Index	Fat (g per svg.)	CHO (g per svg.)
Bran Buds with Psyllium™, Kellogg's, ⅓ cup, 1 oz.	45	1	24
Bran Flakes, Post, ⅔ cup, 1 oz.	74	1	22
Multi-Bran Chex™, General Mills, 1 cup, 2.1 ozs.	58	15	49
Oat bran, 1 tablespoon	55	1	7
Oat bran muffin, 2 ozs.	60	4	28
Rice bran, 1 tablespoon	19	2	5
Breads			
Dark rye, Black bread, 1 slice, 1.7 ozs.	76	1	18
Dark rye, Schinkenbröt, 1 slice, 2 ozs.	86	1	22
French baguette, 1 oz.	95	1	15
Gluten-free bread, 1 slice	90	1	18
Hamburger bun, 1 prepacked bun, 1½ ozs.	61	2	22
Kaiser roll, 1, 2 ozs.	73	2	34
Light deli (American) rye, 1 slice, 1 oz.	68	1	16
Melba toast, 6 pieces, 1 oz.	70	2	23
Natural Ovens 100% Whole Grain, 1 slice, 1.2 ozs.	51	0	17
Natural Ovens Hunger Filler, 1 slice, 1.2 ozs.	59	0	16
Natural Ovens Natural Wheat, 1 slice, 1.2 ozs.	59	0	16
Natural Ovens Happiness, 1 slice, 1.1 oz.	63	0	15
Pita bread, whole wheat, 6½ inch loaf, 2 ozs.	57	2	35
Pumpernickel, whole grain, 1 slice, 1 oz.	51	1	15
Rye bread, 1 slice, 1 oz.	65	1	15
Sourdough, 1 slice, 1½ ozs.	52	1	20
Sourdough rye, Arnold's, 1 slice, 1½ ozs.	57	1	21
White, 1 slice, 1 oz.	70 (av)	1	12
100% stoneground whole wheat, 1 slice, 1½ ozs.	53	1	15
Whole wheat, 1 slice, 1 oz.	69 (av)	1	13
Bread stuffing from mix, 2 ozs.	74	5	13
Breakfast cereals			
All-Bran with extra fiber™, Kellogg's, ½ cup, 1 oz.	51	1	20
Bran Buds with Psyllium™, Kellogg's, ½ cup, 1 oz.	45	1	24
Bran Flakes, Post, ⅔ cup, 1 oz.	74	1	22
Cheerios™, General Mills, 1 cup, 1 oz.	74	2	23
Cocoa Krispies™, Kellogg's, 1 cup, 1 oz.	77	1	27
Corn Bran™, Quaker Crunchy, ¾ cup, 1 oz.	75	1	23
Corn Chex™, Nabisco, 1 cup, 1 oz.	83	0	26
Corn Flakes™, Kellogg's, 1 cup, 1 oz.	84 (av)	0	24
Cream of Wheat, instant, 1 packet, 1 oz.	74	0	21

Food	Glycemic Index	Fat (g per svg.)	CHO (g per svg.)
Cream of Wheat, old fashioned, ¾ cup, cooked, 6 ozs.	66	0	21
Crispix™, Kellogg's, 1 cup, 1 oz.	87	0	25
Frosted Flakes™, Kellogg's, ¾ cup, 1 oz.	55	0	28
Golden Grahams™, General Mills, ¾ cup, 1.6 ozs.	71	1	25
Grapenuts™, Post, ¼ cup, 1 oz.	67	1	27
Grapenuts Flakes™, Post, ¾ cup, 1 oz.	80	1	24
Life™, Quaker, ¾ cup, 1 oz.	66	1	25
Muesli, natural muesli, ⅔ cup, 1½ ozs.	56	3	28
Muesli, toasted, ⅔ cup, 2 ozs.	43	10	41
Multi-Bran Chex™, General Mills, 1 cup, 2.1 ozs.	58	1.5	49
Oat bran, raw, 1 tablespoon	55	1	7
Oat bran™, Quaker Oats, ¾ cup, 1 oz.	50	1	23
Oatmeal (made with water), old fashioned, cooked, ½ cup, 4 ozs.	49 (av)	1	12
Oats, 1-minute, Quaker Oats, 1 cup, cooked	66	2	25
Puffed Wheat™, Quaker, 2 cups, 1 oz.	67	0	22
Raisin Bran™, Kellogg's, ¾ cup, 1 oz.	73	0	32
Rice bran, 1 tablespoon	19	2	5
Rice Chex™, General Mills, 1¼ cups, 1 oz.	89	0	27
Rice Krispies™, Kellogg's, 1¼ cups, 1 oz.	82	0	26
Shredded wheat, spoonsize, ⅔ cup, 1.2 ozs.	58	0	27
Shredded Wheat™, Post, 1 oz.	83	1	23
Smacks™, Kellogg's, ¾ cup, 1 oz.	56	1	24
Special K™, Kellogg's, 1 cup, 1 oz.	66	0	22
Team Flakes™, Nabisco, ¾ cup, 1 oz.	82	0	25
Total™, General Mills, ¾ cup, 1 oz.	76	1	24
Weetabix™, 2 biscuits, 1.2 ozs.	75	1	28
Buckwheat groats, cooked, ½ cup, 2.7 ozs.	54 (av)	1	20
Bulgur, cooked, ⅔ cup, 4 ozs.	48 (av)	0	23
Bun, hamburger, 1 prepacked bun, 1.7 ozs.	61	2	22
Butter beans, boiled, ½ cup, 4 ozs.	31 (av)	0	16
Cakes			
Angel food cake, 1 slice, 1/12 cake, 1 oz.	67	trace	17
Banana bread, 1 slice, 3 ozs.	47	7	46
Pound cake, homemade, 1 slice, 3 ozs.	54	15	42
Sponge cake, 1 slice, 1/12 cake, 2 ozs.	46	4	32
Capellini pasta, cooked, 1 cup, 6 ozs.	45	1	53
Cantaloupe, raw, ¼ small, 6½ ozs.	65	0	16

Food	Glycemic Index	Fat (g per svg.)	CHO (g per svg.)
Carrots, peeled, boiled, canned, ½ cup, 2.4 ozs.	49	0	3
Cereal grains			
Barley, pearled, boiled, ½ cup, 2.6 ozs.	25 (av)	0	22
Bulgur, cooked, ½ cup, 3 ozs.	48 (av)	0	17
Couscous, cooked, ½ cup, 3 ozs.	65 (av)	0	21
Corn			
Cornmeal, whole grain, from mix, cooked, ⅓ cup, 1.4 ozs.	68	1	30
Sweet corn, canned, drained, ½ cup, 3 ozs.	55 (av)	1	15
Taco shells, 2 shells, 1 oz.	68	5	17
Rice			
Basmati, white, boiled, 1 cup, 6 ozs.	58	0	50
Brown, 1 cup, 6 ozs.	55 (av)	0	37
Converted™, Uncle Ben's, 1 cup, 6 ozs.	44	0	38
Instant, cooked, 1 cup, 6 ozs.	87	0	37
Long grain, white, 1 cup, 6 ozs.	56 (av)	0	42
Parboiled, 1 cup, 6 ozs.	48	0	38
Rice cakes, plain, 3 cakes, 1 oz.	82	1	23
Short grain, white, 1 cup, 6 ozs.	72	0	42
Chana dal, ½ cup, 4 ozs.	8	3	28
Cheerios™, General Mills, breakfast cereal, 1 cup, 1 oz.	74	2	23
Cherries, 10 large cherries, 3 ozs.	22	0	10
Chickpeas (garbanzo beans),canned, drained, ½ cup, 4 ozs.	42	2	15
boiled, ½ cup, 3 ozs.	33 (av)	2	23
Chocolate butterscotch muffin, low fat from mix, 1 muffin	53	4	29
Chocolate, bar, 1½ ozs.	49	14	26
Chocolate Flavor, Nestle Quik™ (made with water), 3 teaspoons	53	0	14
Coca-Cola™, soft drink, 1 can	63	0	39
Cocoa Krispies™, Kellogg's, breakfast cereal, 1 cup, 1 oz.	77	1	27
Corn			
Cornmeal, cooked from mix, ⅓ cup, 1.4 ozs.	68	1	30
Sweet corn, canned and drained, ½ cup, 3 ozs.	55 (av)	1	15
Corn Bran™, Quaker Crunchy, breakfast cereal, ¾ cup, 1 oz.	75	1	23
Corn Chex™, General Mills, breakfast cereal, 1 cup, 1 oz.	83	0	26
Corn chips, 1 oz.	72	10	16
Corn Flakes™, Kellogg's, breakfast cereal, 1 cup, 1 oz.	84 (av)	0	24
Cornmeal, from mix, cooked, ⅓ cup, 1.4 ozs.	68	1	30
Cookies			
Graham crackers, 4 squares, 1 oz.	74	3	22

Food	Glycemic Index	Fat (g per svg.)	CHO (g per svg.)
Milk Arrowroot, 3 cookies, ½ oz.	69	2	9
Oatmeal, 1 cookie, ⅔ oz.	55	3	12
Shortbread, 4 small cookies, 1 oz.	64	7	19
Social Tea™ biscuits, Nabisco, 4 cookies, ⅔ oz.	55	3	13
Vanilla wafers, 7 cookies, 1 oz.	77	4	21
see also Crackers			
Couscous, cooked, ⅔ cup, 4 ozs.	65 (av)	0	21
Crackers			
Crispbread, 3 crackers, ⅔ oz.	81	0	15
Kavli™ All Natural Whole Grain Crispbread, 4 wafers, 1 oz.	71	1	16
Premium soda crackers, saltine, 8 crackers, 1 oz.	74	3	17
Rice cakes, plain, 3 cakes, 1 oz.	82	1	23
Ryvita™ Tasty Dark Rye Whole Grain Crisp Bread, 2 slices, ⅔ oz.	69	1	16
Stoned wheat thins, 3 crackers, ⅘ oz.	67	2	15
Water cracker, Carr's, 3 king size crackers, ⅘ oz.	78	2	18
Cream of Wheat, instant, 1 packet, 1 oz.	74	0	21
Cream of Wheat, old fashioned, ¾ cup, cooked, 6 ozs.	66	0	21
Crispix™, Kellogg's, breakfast cereal, 1 cup, 1 oz.	87	0	25
Croissant, medium, 1.2 ozs.	67	14	27
Custard, ½ cup, 4.4 ozs.	43	4	24
Dairy foods and nondairy substitutes			
Ice cream, 10% fat, vanilla, ½ cup, 2.2 ozs.	61 (av)	7	16
Ice milk, vanilla, ½ cup, 2.2 ozs.	50	3	15
Milk, whole, 1 cup, 8 ozs.	27 (av)	9	11
skim, 1 cup, 8 ozs.	32	0	12
chocolate flavored, 1%, 1 cup, 8 ozs.	34	3	26
Pudding, ½ cup, 4.4 ozs.	43	4	24
Soy milk, 1 cup, 8 ozs.	31	7	14
Tofu frozen dessert (nondairy), low fat, ½ cup, 2 ozs.	115	1	21
Yogurt			
nonfat, fruit flavored, with sugar, 8 ozs.	33	0	30
nonfat, plain, artificial sweetener, 8 ozs.	14	0	17
nonfat, fruit flavored, artificial sweetener, 8 ozs.	14	0	16
Dates, dried, 5, 1.4 ozs.	103	0	27
Doughnut with cinnamon and sugar, 1.6 ozs.	76	11	29
Fanta™, soft drink, 1 can	68	0	47
Fava beans, frozen, boiled, ½ cup, 3 ozs.	79	0	17
Fettucine, cooked, 1 cup, 6 ozs.	32	1	57

Food	Glycemic Index	Fat (G PER SVG.)	CHO (G PER SVG.)
Fish sticks, frozen, oven-cooked, fingers, 3½ ozs.	38	14	24
Flan cake, ½ cup, 4 ozs.	65	5	23
French baguette bread, 1 oz.	95	0	15
French fries, large, 4.3 ozs.	75	22	46
Frosted Flakes™, Kellogg's, breakfast cereal, ¾ cup, 1 oz.	55	0	28
Fructose, pure, 3 packets	23 (av)	0	10
Fruit cocktail, canned in natural juice, ½ cup, 4 ozs.	55	0	15
Fruits and fruit products			
Agave nectar (90% fructose syrup), 1 tablespoon	11	0	16
Apple, 1 medium, 5 ozs.	38 (av)	0	18
Apple, dried, 1 oz.	29	0	24
Apple juice, unsweetened, 1 cup, 8 ozs.	40	0	29
Apricots, fresh, 3 medium, 3.3 ozs.	57	0	12
canned, light syrup, 3 halves	64	0	19
dried, 1 oz.	31	0	13
Apricot jam, no added sugar, 1 tablespoon	55	0	17
Banana, raw, 1 medium, 5 ozs.	55 (av)	0	32
Cantaloupe, raw, ¼ small, 6½ ozs.	65	0	16
Cherries, 10 large, 3 ozs.	22	0	10
Dates, dried, 5, 1.4 ozs.	103	0	27
Fruit cocktail, canned in natural juice, ½ cup, 4 ozs.	55	0	15
Grapefruit, raw, ½ medium, 3.3 ozs.	25	0	5
Grapefruit juice, unsweetened, 1 cup, 8 ozs.	48	0	22
Grapes, green, 1 cup, 3 ozs.	46 (av)	0	15
Kiwi, 1 medium, raw, peeled, 2½ ozs.	52 (av)	0	8
Mango, 1 small, 5 ozs.	55 (av)	0	19
Marmalade, 1 tablespoon	48	0	17
Orange, navel, 1 medium, 4 ozs.	44 (av)	0	10
Orange juice, 1 cup, 8 ozs.	46	0	26
Papaya, ½ medium, 5 ozs.	58 (av)	0	14
Peach, fresh, 1 medium, 3 ozs.	28	0	7
canned, natural juice, ½ cup, 4 ozs.	30	0	14
canned, light syrup, ½ cup, 4 ozs.	52	0	18
canned, heavy syrup, ½ cup, 4 ozs.	58	0	26
Pear, fresh, 1 medium, 5 ozs.	38 (av)	0	21
canned in pear juice, ½ cup, 4 ozs.	44	0	13
Pineapple, fresh, 2 slices, 4 ozs.	66	0	10

Food	Glycemic Index	Fat (g per svg.)	CHO (g per svg.)
Pineapple juice, unsweetened, canned, 8 ozs.	46	0	34
Plums, 1 medium, 2 ozs.	39 (av)	0	7
Raisins, ¼ cup, 1 oz.	64	0	28
Strawberry jam, 1 tablespoon	51	0	18
Watermelon, 1 cup, 5 ozs.	72	0	8
Gatorade™ sports drink, 1 cup, 8 ozs.	78	0	14
Glucose powder, 2½ tablets	102	0	10
Gluten-free bread, 1 slice, 1 oz.	90	1	18
Golden Grahams™, General Mills, ¾ cup, 1.6 ozs.	71	1	25
Granola Bars™, Quaker Chewy, 1 oz.	61	2	23
Gnocchi, cooked, 1 cup, 5 ozs.	68	3	71
Graham crackers, 4 squares, 1 oz.	74	3	22
Grapefruit, raw, ½ medium, 3.3 ozs.	25	0	5
Grapefruit juice unsweetened, 1 cup, 8 ozs.	48	0	22
Grapenuts™, Post, breakfast cereal, ¼ cup, 1 oz.	67	1	27
Grapenuts Flakes™, Post, breakfast cereal, ¾ cup, 1 oz.	80	1	24
Grapes, green, 1 cup, 3.3 ozs.	46 (av)	0	15
Green pea soup, canned, ready to serve, 1 cup, 9 ozs.	66	3	27
Hamburger bun, 1 prepacked bun, 1½ ozs.	61	2	22
Honey, 1 tablespoon	58	0	16
Ice cream, 10% fat, vanilla, ½ cup, 2.2 ozs.	61 (av)	7	16
Ice milk, vanilla, ½ cup, 2.2 ozs.	50	3	15
Isostar, 1 cup, 8 ozs.	73	0	18
Jelly beans, 10 large, 1 oz.	80	0	26
Kaiser rolls, 1 roll, 2 ozs.	73	2	34
Kavli™ All Natural Whole Grain Crispbread, 4 wafers, 1 oz.	71	1	16
Kidney beans, red, boiled, ½ cup, 3 ozs.	27 (av)	0	20
Kidney beans, red, canned and drained, ½ cup, 4.3 ozs.	52	0	19
Kiwi, 1 medium, raw, peeled, 2½ ozs.	52 (av)	0	8
Kudos Granola Bars™ (whole grain), 1 bar, 1 oz.	62	5	20
Lactose, pure, ⁷⁄₁₀ oz.	46 (av)	0	10
Lentil soup, Unico, canned, 1 cup, 8 ozs.	44	1	24
Lentils, green and brown, boiled, ½ cup, 3 ozs.	30 (av)	0	16
Lentils, red, boiled, 1.4 cup, 4 ozs.	26 (av)	0	27
Life™, Quaker, breakfast cereal, ¾ cup, 1 oz.	66	1	25
Life Savers™, roll candy, 6 pieces, peppermint	70	0	10
Light deli (American) rye bread, 1 slice, 1 oz.	68	1	16

Food	Glycemic Index	Fat (g per svg.)	CHO (g per svg.)
Lima beans, baby, frozen, ½ cup, 3 ozs.	32	0	17
Linguine pasta, thick, cooked, 1 cup, 6 ozs.	46 (av)	1	56
Linguine pasta, thin, cooked, 1 cup, 6 ozs.	55 (av)	1	56
M&M's Chocolate Candies Peanut™, 1.7 oz. package	33	13	30
Macaroni and Cheese Dinner™, Kraft packaged, cooked, 1 cup, 7 ozs.	64	17	48
Macaroni, cooked, 1 cup, 6 ozs.	45	1	52
Maltose (maltodextrin), pure, 2½ teaspoons	105	0	10
Mango, 1 small, 5 ozs.	55 (av)	0	19
Marmalade, 1 tablespoon	48	0	17
Mars Almond Bar™, 1.8 ozs.	65	12	31
Melba toast, 6 pieces, 1 oz.	70	2	23
Milk, whole, 1 cup, 8 ozs.	27 (av)	9	11
skim, 1 cup, 8 ozs.	32	0	12
chocolate flavored, 1%, 1 cup, 8 ozs.	34	3	26
Milk Arrowroot, 3 cookies, ½ oz.	63	2	9
Millet, cooked, ½ cup, 4 ozs.	71	1	2
Muesli, breakfast cereal, toasted, ⅔ cup, 2 ozs.	43	10	41
Muesli, non-toasted, ⅔ cup, 1½ ozs.	56	3	28
Multi-Bran Chex™, General Mills, 1 cup, 2.1 ozs.	58	1.5	49
Muffins			
Apple cinnamon, from mix, 1 muffin, 2 ozs.	44	8	33
Apricot and honey, low fat, from mix, 1 muffin	60	4	27
Banana, oat and honey, low fat, from mix, 1 muffin	65	4	27
Blueberry, 1 muffin, 2 ozs.	59	4	27
Chocolate butterscotch, low fat, from mix, 1 muffin	53	4	29
Oat and raisin, low fat, from mix, 1 muffin	54	3	28
Oat bran, 1 muffin, 2 ozs.	60	4	28
Mung beans, boiled, ½ cup, 3½ ozs.	38	1	18
Natural Ovens 100% Whole Grain bread, 1 slice, 1.2 ozs.	51	0	17
Natural Ovens Hunger Filler bread, 1 slice, 1.2 ozs.	59	0	16
Natural Ovens Natural Wheat bread, 1 slice, 1.2 ozs.	59	0	16
Natural Ovens Happiness bread, 1 slice, 1.1 ozs.	63	0	15
Navy beans, boiled, ½ cup, 3 ozs.	38 (av)	0	
Nutella™ (spread), 2 tablespoons, 1 oz.	33	9	19
Oat and raisin muffin, low fat from mix, 1 muffin	54	3	28
Oat bran, 1 tablespoon	55	1	7

Food	Glycemic Index	Fat (g per svg.)	CHO (g per svg.)
Oat bran™, Quaker Oats, breakfast cereal, ¾ cup, 1 oz.	50	1	23
Oat bran, 1 muffin, 2 ozs.	60	4	28
Oatmeal (made with water), old fashioned, cooked, 1 cup, 8 ozs.	49	2	26
Oatmeal cookie, 1, ⅔ oz.	55	3	12
Oats, 1-minute, Quaker Oats, 1 cup, cooked	66	2	25
Orange, navel, 1 medium, 4 ozs.	44 (av)	0	10
Orange syrup, diluted, 1 cup	66	0	20
Orange juice, 1 cup, 8 ozs.	46	0	26
Papaya, ½ medium, 5 ozs.	58 (av)	0	14
Parsnips, boiled, ½ cup, 2½ ozs.	97	0	15
Pasta			
Capellini, cooked, 1 cup, 6 ozs.	45	1	53
Fettucine, cooked, 1 cup, 6 ozs.	32	1	57
Gnocchi, cooked, 1 cup, 5 ozs.	68	3	71
Linguine thick, cooked, 1 cup, 6 ozs.	46 (av)	1	56
Linguine thin, cooked, 1 cup, 6 ozs.	55 (av)	1	56
Macaroni, cooked, 1 cup, 5 ozs.	45	1	52
Macaroni & Cheese Dinner™, Kraft, packaged, cooked, 1 cup, 7 ozs.	64	17	48
Ravioli, meat-filled, cooked, 1 cup, 9 ozs.	39	8	32
Spaghetti, white, cooked, 1 cup, 6 ozs.	41 (av)	1	52
Spaghetti, whole wheat, cooked, 1 cup, 6 ozs.	37 (av)	1	48
Spirali, durum, cooked, 1 cup, 6 ozs.	43	1	56
Star Pastina, cooked, 1 cup, 6 ozs.	38	1	56
Tortellini, cheese, cooked, 8 ozs.	50	6	26
Vermicelli, cooked, 1 cup, 6 ozs.	35	0	42
Pastry, flaky, ⅛ of double crust, 2 ozs.	59	15	24
Pea soup, split with ham, canned, 1 cup, Wil-Pak Foods, 5½ ozs.	66	7	56
Peach, fresh, 1 medium, 3 ozs.	28	0	7
canned, heavy syrup, ½ cup, 4 ozs.	58	0	26
canned, light syrup, ½ cup, 4 ozs.	52	0	18
canned, natural juice, ½ cup, 4 ozs.	30	0	14
Peanuts, roasted, salted, ½ cup, 21/2 ozs.	14 (av)	38	16
Pear, fresh, 1 medium, 5 ozs.	38 (av)	0	21
canned in pear juice, ½ cup, 4 ozs.	44	0	13
Peas dried, boiled, ½ cup, 2 ozs.	22	0	7

Food	Glycemic Index	Fat (g per svg.)	CHO (g per svg.)
Pineapple, fresh, 2 slices, 4 ozs.	66	0	10
Pineapple juice, unsweetened, canned, 8 ozs.	46	0	34
Pinto beans, canned, ½ cup, 4 ozs.	45	1	18
Pinto beans, soaked, boiled, ½ cup, 3 ozs.	39	0	22
Pita bread, whole wheat, 6½ inch loaf, 2 ozs.	57	2	35
Pizza, cheese and tomato, 2 slices, 8 ozs.	60	22	56
Plums, 1 medium, 2 ozs.	39 (av)	0	7
Popcorn, light, microwave, 2 cups (popped)	55	3	12
Potatoes			
Desirée, peeled, boiled, 1 medium, 4 ozs.	101	0	13
French fries, large, 4.3 ozs.	75	26	49
instant mashed potatoes, Carnation Foods™, ½ cup, 3½ ozs.	86	2	14
new, unpeeled, boiled, 5 small (cocktail), 6 ozs.	62 (av)	0	23
new, canned, drained, 5 small, 6 ozs.	61	0	23
red-skinned, peeled, boiled, 1 medium, 4 ozs.	88 (av)	0	15
red-skinned, baked in oven (no fat), 1 medium, 4 ozs.	93 (av)	0	15
red-skinned, mashed, ½ cup, 4 ozs.	91 (av)	0	16
red-skinned, microwaved, 1 medium, 4 ozs.	79	0	15
sweet potato, peeled, boiled, ½ cup mashed, 3 ozs.	54 (av)	0	20
white-skinned, peeled, boiled, 1 medium, 4 ozs.	63 (av)	0	24
white-skinned, with skin, baked in oven (no fat), 1 medium, 4 ozs.	85 (av)	0	30
white-skinned, mashed, ½ cup, 4 ozs.	70 (av)	0	20
white-skinned, with skin, microwaved, 1 medium, 4 ozs.	82	0	29
Sebago, peeled, boiled, 1 medium, 4 ozs.	87	0	13
Potato chips, plain, 14 pieces, 1 oz.	54 (av)	11	15
Pound cake, 1 slice, homemade, 3 ozs.	54	15	42
Power Bar™, Performance, Chocolate, 1 bar	58	2	45
Premium saltine crackers, 8 crackers, 1 oz.	74	3	17
Pretzels, 1 oz.	83	1	22
Puffed Wheat™, Quaker, breakfast cereal, 2 cups, 1 oz.	67	0	22
Pumpernickel bread, whole grain, 2 slices	51	2	30
Pumpkin, peeled, boiled, mashed, ½ cup, 4 ozs.	75	0	6
Raisins, ¼ cup, 1 oz.	64	0	28
Raisin Bran™, Kellogg's, breakfast cereal, ¾ cup, 1.3 ozs.	73	0	32
Ravioli, meat-filled, cooked, 1 cup, 9 ozs.	39	8	32

Food	Glycemic Index	Fat (g per svg.)	CHO (g per svg.)
Rice			
Basmati, white, boiled, 1 cup, 7 ozs.	58	0	50
Brown, 1 cup, 6 ozs.	55 (av)	0	37
Converted™, Uncle Ben's, 1 cup, 6 ozs.	44	0	38
Instant, cooked, 1 cup, 6 ozs.	87	0	37
Long grain, white, 1 cup, 6 ozs.	56 (av)	0	42
Parboiled, 1 cup, 6 ozs.	48	0	38
Rice bran, 1 tablespoon	19	2	5
Rice cakes, plain, 3 cakes, 1 oz.	82	1	23
Short grain, white, 1 cup, 6 ozs.	72	0	42
Rice Chex™, General Mills, breakfast cereal, 1¼ cups, 1 oz.	89	0	27
Rice Krispies™, Kellogg's, breakfast cereal, 1¼ cups, 1 oz.	82	0	26
Rice vermicelli, cooked, 6 ozs.	58	0	48
Roll (bread), Kaiser, 1 roll, 2 ozs.	73	2	39
Romano (cranberry) beans, boiled, ½ cup, 3 ozs.	46	0	21
Rutabaga, peeled, boiled, ½ cup, 2.6 ozs.	72	0	3
Rye bread, 1 slice, 1 oz.	65	1	15
Ryvita™ Tasty Dark Rye Whole Grain Crisp Bread, 2 slices, ⅔ oz.	69	1	16
Sausages, smoked link, pork and beef, fried, 2½ oz.	28	29	5
Semolina, cooked, ⅔ cup, 6 ozs.	55	0	17
Shortbread, 4 small cookies, 1 oz.	64	7	19
Shredded Wheat™, Post, breakfast cereal, 1 oz.	83	1	23
Shredded wheat, 1 biscuit, ⅙ oz.	62	0	19
Skittles Original Fruit Bite Size Candies™, 2.3 oz. pk.	70	3	59
Smacks™, Kellogg's, breakfast cereal, ¾ cup, 1 oz.	56	1	24
Snickers™, 2.2 oz. bar	41	15	36
Social Tea™ biscuits, Nabisco, 4 cookies, ⅔ oz.	55	3	13
Soft drink, Fanta™, 1 can, 12 ozs.	68	0	47
Soups			
Black bean soup, ½ cup, 4½ ozs.	64	2	19
Green pea soup, canned, ready to serve, 1 cup, 9 ozs.	66	3	27
Lentil soup, Unico, canned, 1 cup, 8 ozs.	44	1	24
Pea soup, split, with ham, Wil-Pak Foods, 1 cup, 5½ ozs.	66	7	56
Tomato soup, canned, 1 cup, 9 ozs.	38	4	33
Sourdough bread, 1 slice, 1½ ozs.	52	1	20
Rye bread, Arnold's, 1 slice, 1½ ozs.	57	1	21
Soy beans, boiled, ½ cup, 3 ozs.	18 (av)	7	10

Food	Glycemic Index	Fat (g per svg.)	CHO (g per svg.)
Soy milk, 1 cup, 8 ozs.	31	7	14
Spaghetti, white, cooked, 1 cup	41 (av)	1	52
Spaghetti, whole wheat, cooked, 1 cup, 5 ozs.	37 (av)	1	48
Special K™, Kellogg's, breakfast cereal, 1 cup, 1 oz.	66	0	22
Spirali, durum, cooked, 1 cup, 6 ozs.	43	1	56
Split pea soup, 8 ozs.	60	4	38
Split peas, yellow, boiled, ½ cup, 3½ ozs.	32	0	21
Sponge cake plain, 1 slice, 3 ½ ozs.	46	4	32
Sports drinks			
Gatorade™ 1 cup, 8 ozs.	78	0	14
Isostar, 1 cup, 8 ozs.	73	0	18
Sportsplus, 1 cup, 8 ozs.	74	0	17
Sports bars			
Power Bar™, Performance Chocolate Bar, 1 bar	58	2	45
Stoned wheat thins, 3 crackers, ⅙ oz.	67	2	15
Strawberry Nestle Quik™ (made with water), 3 teaspoons	64	0	14
Strawberry jam, 1 tablespoon	51	0	18
Sucrose, 1 teaspoon	65 (av)	0	4
Syrup, fruit flavored, diluted, 1 cup	66	0	20
Sweet corn, canned, drained, ½ cup, 3 ozs.	55 (av)	1	16
Sweet potato, peeled, boiled, ½ cup mashed, 3 ozs.	54 (av)	0	20
Taco shells, 2 shells, 1 oz.	68	5	17
Tapioca pudding, boiled with whole milk, 1 cup, 10 ozs.	81	13	51
Taro, peeled, boiled, ½ cup, 2 ozs.	54	0	23
Team Flakes™, Nabisco, breakfast cereal, ¾ cup, 1 oz.	82	0	25
Tofu frozen dessert, nondairy, low fat, 2 ozs.	115	1	21
Tomato soup, canned, 1 cup, 9 ozs.	38	4	33
Tortellini, cheese, cooked, 8 ozs.	50	6	26
Total™, General Mills, breakfast cereal, ¾ cup, 1 oz.	76	1	24
Twix Chocolate Caramel Cookie™, 2, 2 ozs.	44	14	37
Vanilla wafers, 7 cookies, 1 oz.	77	4	21
Vermicelli, cooked, 1 cup, 6 ozs.	35	0	42
Vitasoy™ Soy milk, creamy original, 1 cup, 8 ozs.	31	7	14
Waffles, plain, frozen, 4 inch square, 1 oz.	76	3	13
Water crackers, 3 king size crackers, ⅚ oz.	78	2	18
Watermelon, 1 cup, 5 ozs.	72	0	8
Weetabix™ breakfast cereal, 2 biscuits, 1.2 ozs.	75	1	28

Food	Glycemic Index	Fat (g per svg.)	CHO (g per svg.)
White bread, 1 slice, 1 oz.	70 (av)	1	12
Whole wheat bread, 1 slice, 1 oz.	69 (av)	1	13
Yam, boiled, 3 ozs.	51	0	31
Yogurt			
nonfat, fruit flavored, with sugar, 8 ozs.	33	0	30
nonfat, plain, artificial sweetener, 8 ozs.	14	0	17
nonfat, fruit flavored, artificial sweetener, 8 ozs.	14	0	16

GLYCEMIC INDEX TESTING

If you are a food manufacturer, you may be interested in having the glycemic index of some of your products tested on a fee-for-service basis. For more information, contact either:

Glycaemic Index Testing Inc.
135 Mavety Street
Toronto, Ontario
Canada M6P 2L8
E-mail: thomas.wolever@utoronto.ca

or

Sydney University Glycaemic Index Research Service (SUGIRS)
Department of Biochemistry
University of Sydney
NSW 2006 Australia
Fax: (61) (2) 9351-6022
E-mail: j.brandmiller@staff.usyd.edu.au

FOR MORE INFORMATION

REGISTERED DIETITIANS

Registered Dietitians (R.D.s) are nutrition experts who provide sports nutrition assessment and guidance. Check for the initials "R.D." after the name to identify qualified dietitians who provide the highest standard of care to their clients. Glycemic index is part of their training so all dietitians should be able to help in applying the principles in this guide, but some dietitians do specialize in certain areas. If you want more detailed advice on sports nutrition and the glycemic index just ask the dietitian whether this is a specialty when you make your appointment.

Dietitians work in hospitals and often run their own private practices as well. For a list of dietitians in your area, contact the American Dietetic Association (ADA) Consumer Nutrition Hotline (1-800-366-1655) or visit ADA's home page at the address below. You can also check the Yellow Pages under "Dietitians."

The American Dietetic Association
216 West Jackson Boulevard
Chicago, IL 60606
Phone: 1-800-877-1600
Fax: 1-312-899-1979
Web site: http://www.eatright.org/

NATURAL OVENS ORDERING INFORMATION

Natural Ovens of Manitowoc
4300 County Trunk CR
P.O. Box 730
Manitowoc WI 54221-073
Telephone: 1-800-772-0730
Fax: 920-758-2594
http://www.naturalovens.com/

ACKNOWLEDGMENTS

We would like to acknowledge the extraordinary efforts of Johanna Burani and Linda Rao, who adapted this book—and the other books in *The Glucose Revolution Pocket Guide* series—for North American readers. Together they have worked to ensure that every piece of information is accurate and appropriate for readers in the U.S. and Canada.

ABOUT THE AUTHORS

Helen O'Connor, B.Sc., Dip. N.D., Ph.D., is an accredited dietitian specializing in sports nutrition. She obtained her Ph.D. in the Department of Medicine, University of Sydney and now works in the Department of Exercise and Sport Science lecturing in exercise biochemistry and sports nutrition. She is also the consultant to the New South Wales Institute of Sport where she works with elite athletes, assisting them with their dietary needs. A consultant to two professional football teams and the president of Sports Dietitians Australia, she has published five books on sports nutrition.

Jennie Brand-Miller, Ph.D., Associate Professor of Human Nutrition in the Human Nutrition Unit, Department of Biochemistry, University of Sydney, Australia, is widely recognized as one of the world's leading authorities on the glycemic index. She received her B.Sc. (1975) and Ph.D. (1979) degrees from the Department of Food Science and Technology at the University of New South Wales, Australia. She is the editor of the *Proceedings of the Nutrition Society of Australia* and a member of the Scientific Consultative Committee of the Australian Nutrition Foundation. She has written more than 200 research papers, including 60 on the glycemic index of foods. A co-author of *The Glucose*

Revolution and all the titles in *The Glucose Revolution Pocket Guide* Series, she lives in Sydney, Australia.

Thomas M. S. Wolever, M.D., Ph.D., another of the world's leading authorities of the glycemic index, is Professor in the Department of Nutritional Sciences, University of Toronto, and a member of the Division of Endocrinology and Metabolism, St. Michael's Hospital, Toronto. He is a graduate of Oxford University (B.A., M.A., M.B., B.Ch., M.Sc., and D.M.). He received his Ph.D. at the University of Toronto. His research since 1980 has focused on the glycemic index of foods and the prevention of type 2 diabetes. A co-author of *The Glucose Revolution* and all the titles in *The Glucose Revolution Pocket Guide* Series, he lives in Toronto, Canada.

Stephen Colagiuri, M.D., is the President of the Australian Diabetes Society, director of the Diabetes Center, and head of the Department of Endocrinology, Metabolism, and Diabetes at the Prince of Wales Hospital, Randwick, New South Wales, Australia. He is a graduate of the University of Sydney (M.B.B.S., 1970) and a member of the Royal Australasian College of Physicians (1977). He has joint academic appointments at the University of New South Wales. He has authored more than 100 scientific papers, many concerned with the importance of carbohydrate in the diet of people with diabetes. A co-author of *The Glucose Revolution* and several other titles in *The Glucose Revolution Pocket Guide* Series, he lives in Sydney, Australia.

Kaye Foster-Powell, B.Sc., M. Nutr. & Diet, is an accredited dietitian-nutritionist in both public and private practice in New South Wales, Australia. A graduate of the University of Sydney (B.Sc., 1987; Masters of Nutrition and Dietetics, 1994), she has extensive experience in diabetes management and has researched practical applications of the glycemic index over the last 5 years. A co-author of *The Glucose Revolution* and all the titles in *The Glucose Revolution Pocket Guide* Series, she lives in Sydney, Australia.

Johanna Burani, M.S., R.D., C.D.E., is a registered dietitian and certified diabetes educator with more than 10 years experience in nutritional counseling. She specializes in designing individual meal plans based on low glycemic-index food choices. The adapter of *The Glucose Revolution* and co-adapter, with Linda Rao, of all the titles in *The Glucose Revolution Pocket Guide* Series, she is the author of seven books and professional manuals, and lives in Mendham, New Jersey.

Linda Rao, M.Ed., a freelance writer and editor, has been writing and researching health topics for the past 11 years. Her work has appeared in several national publications, including *Prevention* and *USA Today*. She serves as a contributing editor for *Prevention* Magazine and is the co-adapter, with Johanna Burani, of all the titles in *The Glucose Revolution Pocket Guide* Series. She lives in Allentown, Pennsylvania.

The Glucose Revolution begins here . . .

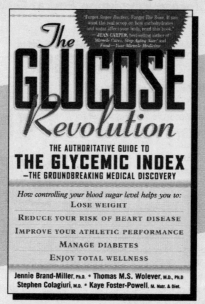

THE GLUCOSE REVOLUTION
The Authoritative Guide to the Glycemic Index—
The Groundbreaking Medical Discovery

National Bestseller!

"Forget *Sugar Busters*. Forget *The Zone*. If you want the real scoop on how carbohydrates and sugar affect your body, read this book by the world's leading researchers on the subject. It's the authoritative, last word on choosing foods to control your blood sugar."

—Jean Carper, best-selling author of *Miracle Brain, Miracle Cures, Stop Aging Now!* and *Food—Your Miracle Medicine*

ISBN 1-56924-660-2 • $14.95

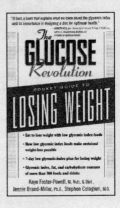
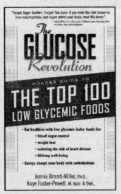

The Glucose Revolution Pocket Guide to
DIABETES

Help control your diabetes with low glycemic index foods

Based on the most up-to-date information about carbohydrates, this basic guide to the glycemic index and diabetes allows people with type 1 and type 2 diabetes to make more informed choices about their diets. Topics covered include why many traditionally "taboo" foods don't cause the unfavorable effects on blood sugar levels they were believed to have, and why diets based on low G.I. foods improve blood sugar control. Also covered are how to include more of the right kinds of carbohydrates in your diet, the

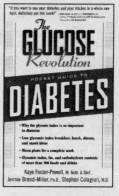

optimum diet for people with diabetes, practical hints for meal preparation and tips to help make the glycemic index work throughout the day, a week of low G.I. menus, G.I. success stories, and more.

ISBN 1-56924-675-0 • $4.95

The Glucose Revolution Pocket Guide to
SUGAR AND ENERGY

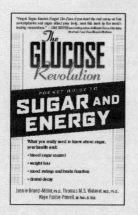

Sugar's off the black list—find out why

Based on the most up-to-date information about carbohydrates, this basic guide to the glycemic index dispels many common myths about sugar and why it's high time to get rid of the guilt. With evidence showing that restricting refined sugar in your diet may do more harm than good, the authors show you how to intelligently give in to your sugar cravings and regulate your sugar intake to control your blood sugar level and lose weight, with the glycemic index for nearly 150 foods.

ISBN 1-56924-641-6 • $4.95
Forthcoming June 2000

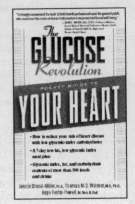